EXTERNAL INFECTIONS OF THE EYE

Bacterial, Viral, and Mycotic

SECOND EDITION

Helena Biantovskaya Fedukowicz

Formerly Adjunct Associate Professor of Clinical Ophthalmology
New York University School of Medicine
New York, New York;
Head of the Microbiology Laboratory
Department of Ophthalmology
Bellevue Hospital
New York, New York

Contributions by
Robert A. Hyndiuk
Sam Seideman

Illustrated by
Beatrice Grover

Forewords by
Goodwin M. Breinin

APPLETON-CENTURY-CROFTS/New York

78 79 80 81 82 / 10 9 8 7 6 5 4 3 2 1

Prentice-Hall International, Inc., London
Prentice-Hall of Australia, Pty. Ltd., Sydney
Prentice-Hall of India Private Limited, New Delhi
Prentice-Hall of Japan, Inc., Tokyo
Prentice-Hall of Southeast Asia (Pte.) Ltd., Singapore
Whitehall Books Ltd., Wellington, New Zealand

Library of Congress Cataloging in Publication Data

Fedukowicz, Helena Biantovskaya.
External infections of the eye, second edition

Includes bibliographies and index.
    1. Eye—Infections. 2. Eye—Microbiology.
I. Hyndiuk, Robert A., joint author. II. Seideman,
Sam, joint author. III. Title. [DNLM: 1. Eye
diseases. 2. Bacterial infections. 3. Virus
diseases. 4. Mycoses. WW100 F294e]
RE96.F4 1977   617.7'1   77-24287
ISBN 0-8385-2322-6

Text design: Joann Berg
Cover design: Kristin Herzog

EXTERNAL INFECTIONS
OF THE EYE

*This book is dedicated
to students
all over the world*

Contributors

Robert A. Hyndiuk, M.D.
Professor of Ophthalmology
Medical College of Wisconsin
Milwaukee, Wisconsin;
Director Cornea-External Disease Unit
The Eye Institute
Milwaukee County Medical Complex
Milwaukee, Wisconsin

Sam Seideman, M.D.
Ophthalmology Staff
Central Vermont Medical Center
Montpelier, Vermont

Contents

Preface

The great progress and advances in the knowledge of microbiology and increasing requests for the original edition, which has been sold out, created a necessity for a new edition. As in the original edition, the importance of a basic approach is emphasized.

Several chapters have been revised and rewritten with outdated material changed and new information added. The additional chapter, Clinical and Laboratory Techniques in External Diseases and Endophthalmitis, contributed by Dr. Robert Hyndiuk, is a timely and welcome inclusion.

Some bacterial nomenclatures have been changed in accordance with the eighth edition of Bergey's *Manual of Determinative Microbiology.*

The cytologic study of conjunctival and corneal scrapings has been extended and its diagnostic importance emphasized. Many color illustrations have been added.

The references are considerable and are historically significant as well as bringing the book up to date. This bibliography may serve to introduce the reader to a more comprehensive study of the subject.

The second edition, like the first, is directed to students and practicing ophthalmologists. Hopefully, it provides a compact, concise, easily read presentation of those problems of eye infections which are of the greatest practical importance. It is hoped that this edition will be even more useful in improving clinical diagnoses, choice of treatment, and teaching purposes. The author is pleased to report that the first edition is widely used in the United States and abroad.

In addition to those mentioned in the first edition, I also wish to thank Mr. R. Newman for his skilled microphotography: he is one of the rare specialists in this field of ophthalmology. My deep gratitude to M. R. Allansmith for revising the chapter on immunology. I thank Drs. H. J. Kaufman, S. A. Rosenthal, S. Stenson, and M. Spinack for their kindness in supplying many interesting slides. I also wish to acknowledge those ophthalmologists, microbiologists, and micologists who gave valuable assistance and suggestions.

My warmest thanks to Mrs. J. Rolls who gave devoted service with skill and patience to transcribe this difficult manuscript into a clear and intelligible work.

My gratitude is also extended to Appleton-Century-Crofts for their accurate skilled work and helpful suggestions in preparing this book.

We are grateful to the Hearst Foundation for partial support of the preparation of the manuscript and illustrations.

Helena Biantovskaya Fedukowicz

Preface to the First Edition

"One careful observation is worth a thousand alibis."

A modern English treatise on ocular infections including laboratory diagnosis and treatment does not exist. In this day of refined technic and instrumentation, the basic approach to disease and diagnosis has been mislaid. It is my intention to provide not only a reference book on ophthalmic bacteriology, virology, mycology, and cytology but also a practical guide to the study of external ocular diseases.

This book deals primarily with the infectious diseases of the external ocular structures. The more common disease entities are stressed. An approach to understanding the entire disease process and not only the fait accompli (ie, the end stage of a disease) is attempted. Not only are the biologic characteristics of the offending organisms discussed but also the host characteristics and responses. Each chapter begins with a description of basic general principles. Specific clinical and laboratory findings are then described and correlated. Predisposing factors including age, nutrition, climate, and hygiene are mentioned, for they are important in planning treatment.

Diagnostic methods have been simplified so that they may be used even by the busy practitioner. The therapeutic measures mentioned have been chosen because I have found them to be effective.

References are given at the end of each chapter. Some have historical value. Most others are of recent origin and were gathered primarily from the English language literature.

The practicality of this book is enhanced by numerous illustrations. These with few exceptions are original. Some photographs have been retouched, and some of the paintings have details exaggerated for purposes of emphasis.

The material for the book was developed in the Department of Ophthalmology of the New York University School of Medicine. Thousands of cases of external disease, including those from other clinics and private practice in New York City, have been studied in the laboratory by smear, scraping, and culture, as well as sensitivity and biochemical tests. Records of all these cases were consulted and used in the preparation of this book. The ophthalmic terminology of Duke-Elder is mainly used. I hope that this book will stimulate both students and practicing ophthalmologists to apply basic knowledge and simple laboratory methods to improve diagnosis and treatment of eye infections.

It is impossible to give full acknowledgment for all the help I have received while working on this text. I feel strongly that this book is a collective effort: that of colleagues, students, laboratory workers, librarians, secretaries, and especially of Beatrice Grover, who illustrated the book, and Katherine Sanborn West, who worked closely with me in editing the manuscript. Had either of them faltered during the years of our working together, I could not have finished this book.

I also wish to express deep gratitude to the late Mrs. Antoinette Peterson, who gave indispensable aid in establishing me in my new country.

My profound thanks to:

Dr. Goodwin M. Breinin, Head of the Department of Ophthalmology, for approving the project, reading the manuscript, and for creating the conditions in which our work could be done.

Dr. A. Gerard DeVoe for encouraging and goading me into undertaking the writing.

Dr. Phillips Thygeson for his critical evaluation which led to many helpful changes and additions to the manuscript.

Dr. Alson E. Braley for making this book possible by giving me my first medical appointment in this country.

Dr. George N. Wise for being my good friend and severest critic and spurring me on to make this book better than I knew how.

Dr. Paul Henkind for giving his precious time to help me achieve whatever special qualities this text may have.

Dr. Benjamin Mandel for his valuable criticism of the section on viral infections.

Miss Beatrice Toharsky for her constant availability for consultation, and for her criticism of individual sections on bacterial infections.

Mr. William C. Porth for his immediate understanding and assistance.

Mrs. Joyce Rolls for being a constant source of help in times of stress.

The publisher and editorial staff for exceptional interest and encouragement.

Mr. Walter Lentschner, a photographer of great experience and skill, for producing all the photographs.

The Albert and Mary Lasker Foundation, Allen Grover, and an anonymous donor for their understanding of the educational need for the book and for their generosity in providing funds for the color plates.

Helena Biantovskaya Fedukowicz

Foreword

The second edition of this standard textbook of ophthalmic bacteriology and external disease by Dr. Fedukowicz should be warmly welcomed by the profession. The enthusiastic and widespread acceptance of the first edition attested to its overall excellence. In the second edition the author has extensively revised many of the chapters and added much material. There are additional discussions of the mimeae organisms, serratia, "anonymous" mycobacteria and others.

The TRIC diseases are herein described as a chlamidial group instead of large viruses. There are additional data on the Herpes viruses as well as adeno and other viruses. The cytology of conjunctival and corneal scrapings is further developed as an important diagnostic method, accompanied by new colored illustrations. The New York University laboratory was a pioneer in the development of the routine practice of cytologic diagnoses.

A chapter on clinical and laboratory techniques by Drs. Robert Hyndiuk and Sam Seideman is a welcomed addition to this volume.

It is my belief that the second edition of this textbook will achieve an even wider distribution and should prove an important aid to students and practitioners of ophthalmology.

Goodwin M. Breinin

Foreword to the First Edition

Dr. Fedukowicz has presented the practitioner, resident, and student of ophthalmology with an integrated textbook of external diseases and microbiology of the eye. I can think of few areas in ophthalmology where the need has been as pressing. The author brings to this study the experiences of thirteen years as Director of the Laboratory of Ophthalmic Bacteriology at New York University School of Medicine and Bellevue Hospital. Her many years as a practicing ophthalmologist in Europe are reflected in a synthesis of the viewpoints of ophthalmologist and laboratory investigator. Furthermore, a long experience in teaching medical students and residents has enabled the author to present the essentials of this subject in a clear and graphic text.

The unified color plates of clinical, bacteriologic, and cytologic data, embellished by Mrs. Grover's artistry, should prove exceedingly useful to all workers in ophthalmology.

Goodwin M. Breinin

Plates 1–47

Plate 1

1. Chronic ulcerative blepharitis due to staphylococci. Ulcers at roots of lashes are covered by dry crusts. The process may last for years. Avoid over-treatment. Antibiotics to be chosen according to sensitivity test. Remove crusts before taking specimen; use wet saline swab. Smear and culture are necessary.

2. Hordeolum internum (meibomitis) due to staphylococci. This condition is often associated with blepharitis; it may be multiple and recurrent. Characterized by pain and localized swelling. A yellow spot is usually seen through the conjunctiva. Preauricular glands are often enlarged.

3. Catarrhal marginal ulcer of cornea, the usual consequence of staphylococcal blepharoconjunctivitis. Single or several superficial infiltrates are separated from the limbus by a clear zone. Infiltrates easily ulcerate. No bacteria are found. The condition is regarded as allergic or toxic.

4. Acute purulent conjunctivitis due to staphylococci. Palpebral conjunctiva, especially of lower lid, is usually involved. Acute process often becomes chronic, with associated blepharitis.

5. Varied morphology of staphylococci. **A.** Staphylococci from panophthalmitis (scraping, Giemsa stain). Unusual, intracellular, kidney-shaped diplococci predominate (can be confused with gonococci). Culture and gram stain confirm diagnosis. Note neutrophils. **B.** Staphylococci from blepharoconjunctivitis (smear, gram stain). May be diagnosed in direct smear by round shape, regular size, and clusterlike arrangement. Culture is needed for pathogenicity and sensitivity tests and to confirm diagnosis.

6. Cultures of *Staphylococcus*. Colonies are circular, discrete, elevated, opaque, and glistening.

2

Plate   1

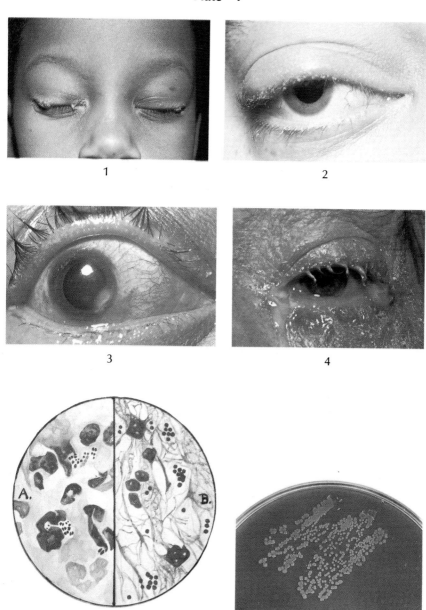

Plate 2

1. Chronic blepharitis. This process is of long duration. Observe the thickening of lid margins (tylosis ciliaris); also note that only a few atrophic cilia remain (madarosis).

2. Sebaceous cyst (atheroma). Considered to be a retention cyst, this may grow to considerable size. The usual location is the inner canthus, which may cause confusion with dacryocystitis. Staphylococci are isolated.

3. Coagulase test. A slide with two drops of bacterial emulsion. The dark area on each shows where human plasma has been added. White spots indicate coagulation. **A.** Negative. **B.** Positive.

4.. Mannitol fermentation. Yellow tube shows change of color from pink to yellow due to *S. aureus*. Test negative in *S. epidermidis*.

5. Disk sensitivity test. This shows a resistant strain of *Staphylococcus*, obviously sensitive to albamycin and slightly to chloromycetin.

6. Varied morphology of staphylococci (smear from culture). **A.** From panophthalmitis. Among typical round cocci are a few kidney-shaped staphylococci. **B.** From blepharitis. Illustrates typical morphology: round shape, regularity of size and staining, and clusterlike arrangement.

4

Plate 2

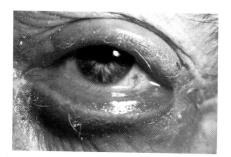

1

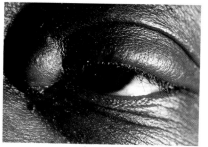

2

A B

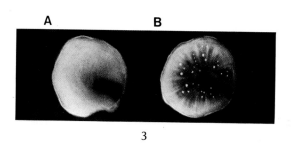

3

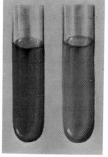

4

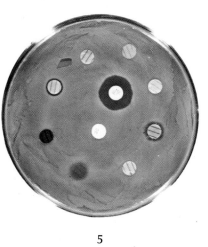

5

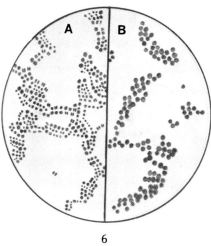

6

Plate 3

1. Pneumococcal acute mucopurulent conjunctivitis. Most frequent type of acute bacterial conjunctivitis. Moderate severity; mild mucopurulent exudation. Pronounced redness of bulbar conjunctiva; petechiae (frequent on upper bulbar conjunctiva; rarely found on lower). Note follicles in lower fornix. Marginal or punctate keratitis may occur.

2. Pneumococcal hypopyon ulcer (serpiginous type). Beginning stage of purulent, very destructive keratitis. This may result in perforation and panophthalmitis. Infection is usually secondary to corneal abrasion. The condition is often associated with chronic dacryocystitis. Hypopyon is sterile and indicates acute iritis. The progressive margin is undermined. Take specimen from this pocket, by loop.

3. Granulomatous masses following acute suppurative dacryocystitis.

4. Acute suppurative dacryocystitis. Pus discharged from opening (fistula), typically below lacrimal sac. The pneumococcus is the most common pathogen.

5. Exudate (original smear) from acute pneumococcal conjunctivitis, illustrating encapsulated lancet-shaped diplococci. Eosinophilic cell may indicate an allergic reaction to infection.

6. Neonatal dacryocystitis. The exudate in the beginning is sterile (often overlooked). Later infections, such as staphylococcus, pneumococcus, haemophilus bacilli, and others, can follow.

Plate 3

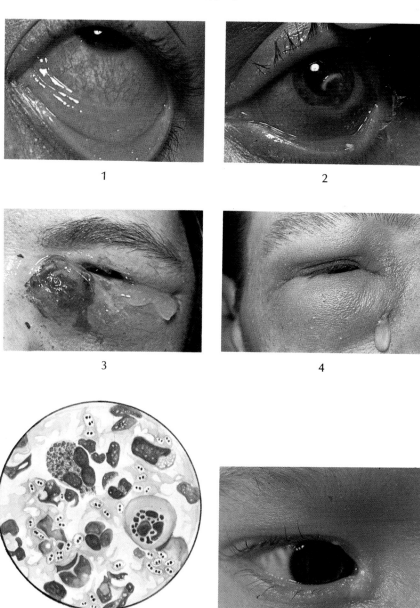

1

2

3

4

5

6

Plate 4

1. Capsule stain (Hiss copper sulfate method). Heavy, unstained capsule seen against violet background.

2. Pneumococci from blood agar culture. Morphology differs from that in the original smear; here, the pneumococci are irregular in size. Note the distinct capsule, which differentiates the pneumococcus from alpha streptococci.

3. Optochin sensitivity test. Place the optochin disk on a blood agar culture of pneumococci. Unlike alpha streptococci, it shows a zone of inhibition indicating sensitivity to optochin. **A.** Pneumococcus. **B.** Alpha streptococci.

4. Culture of pneumococci on blood agar. Tiny, glistening colonies, surrounded by a green zone of incomplete alpha hemolysis (indistinguishable from alpha streptococci).

5. Bile solubility test to differentiate streptococcus from the pneumococcus. Tube on right, with opaque appearance, demonstrates insolubility of alpha streptococci. Clear, transparent contents of tube at left indicate solubility of *S. pneumoniae* (pneumococci).

Plate 4

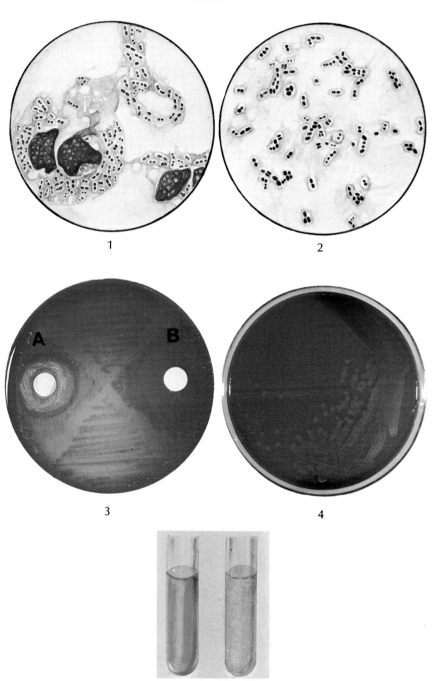

1

2

3

4

5

Plate 5

1. Endophthalmitis bordering on panophthalmitis due to *S. alpha* (viridans, pyogenic, mitis).

2. Central hypopyon ulcer *(S. alpha)*. This may be more severe than pneumococcal ulcer.

3. Posterior abscess due to *S. pyogenes*. This condition is rare, found in extremely virulent infection. Exudate in posterior layers of cornea. Descemet's membrane bulges and may rupture into anterior chamber.

4. Morphologic characteristics of alpha streptococci. **A.** Original exudate from hypopyon ulcer (gram stain). Elongated cocci in diplo or short chain arrangement. No capsule. **B.** Smear from Brewer's culture. In fluid medium, long chains develop.

5. Culture of alpha streptococci on blood agar is similar to pneumococcal culture; the colonies are small, flat, and surrounded by a green zone of incomplete alpha hemolysis.

Plate   5

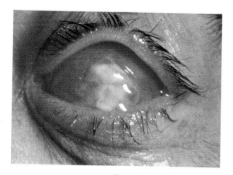

1

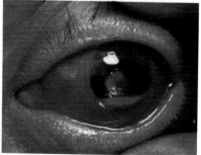

2

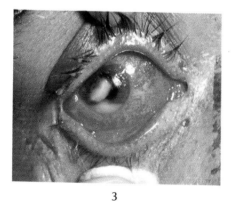

3

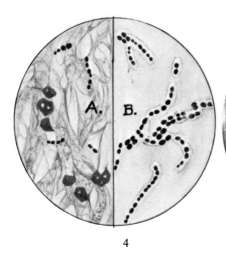

4

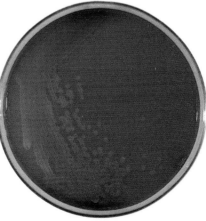

5

Plate 6

1. True membranous conjunctivitis due to *S. pyogenes* (beta). Coagulative fibrinous exudate, penetrating interepithelial spaces and subepithelial tissue, forms a heavy membrane. Unlike *C. diphtheriae*, the membrane may develop on bulbar conjunctiva also.

2. Dramatic destructive beta streptococcal keratitis characterized by profuse, fibrinous, purulent exudate and rapid necrosis of the cornea.

3. *S. pyogenes* culture on blood agar. Important characteristics; small, pointed, opaque colonies surrounded by a big zone (2 to 4 mm or extended area) of complete beta hemolysis.

4. *S. pyogenes* in smear from culture (gram stain). Diplococci or short chain arrangement found in culture on solid medium (blood agar). The same streptococcus shows long chains in fluid medium (Brewer).

5. Cellulitis of the upper lid due to *S. pyogenes*. A history of injury is usual. Process in late stage shows extensive sloughing due to necrosis. The cornea is not involved. The preauricular node is not enlarged. Consequences may be heavy scarring, ectropion, or lagophthalmos.

6. Panophthalmitis due to *S. pyogenes*. All structures of the eye show suppurative inflammation. Tremendous chemosis, swelling, and redness of lids. Infiltration of Tenon's capsule causes exophthalmos.

Plate 6

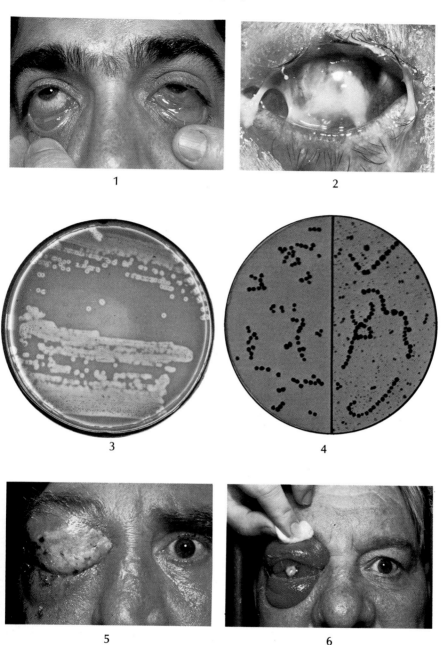

1

2

3

4

5

6

Plate 7

1. *C. xerosis* in scraping (Giemsa stain). *C. xerosis* is the most frequent and most confusing organism found in the eye. Often gives diplococcal appearance (when metachromatic granules present at poles). Important characteristics: uninterrupted wall, irregular size and shape, no capsule, and found on degenerated keratinized epithelium.

2. *C. xerosis* in smears from culture on blood agar (showing variety of morphology). Irregularities of size and shape (club-shaped bodies), V, L, and palisade arrangement are important clues.

3. Bitot's spot. Foamy white, dry, lusterless spot localized in temporal or nasal interpalpebral zone of bulbar conjunctiva. Condition often associated with night blindness. Scraping shows keratinized epithelium containing numerous *C. xerosis* bacilli.

4. Keratomalacia. Usually occurs in children. The condition causes complete destruction of the cornea, associated with debility and malnutrition. *C. xerosis* bacilli are invariably present in large numbers.

5. *C. xerosis* culture on blood agar. **A.** Dustlike, opaque colonies with dry appearance. Growth is slow (two to seven days). **B.** Culture with unusually dry, crusted appearance. *C. xerosis* alone was identified. Isolated from a Puerto Rican patient with an old trachoma.

6. Metachromatic granules (Neisser stain). Important indication for differential diagnosis; limited number of dark metachromatic granules distributed throughout the body of *C. xerosis*.

Plate   7

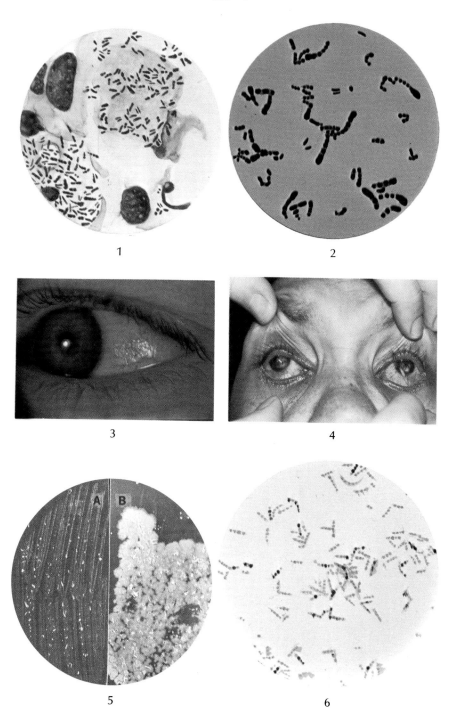

1

2

3

4

5

6

Plate 8

1. Diphtheritic membranous conjunctivitis. Membrane develops on tarsal conjunctiva. It is composed of yellowish gray, coagulated necrotic material embedded in exuded fibrin. Interepithelial spaces and subepithelial tissue are penetrated. When membrane is removed, bleeding occurs. Conjunctivitis may be complicated by severe purulent keratitis.

2. Diphtheritic mucopurulent conjunctivitis. Indistinguishable from other bacterial conjunctivitides. Characterized by mucopurulent discharge without true membrane.

3. Metachromatic granules of C. *diphtheriae* (Neisser stain). Granules are moderate in number and located at poles, giving a drumstick appearance. Cultures and virulence test are needed for diagnosis.

4. C. *diphtheriae* cultures. **A.** Tellurite medium. Intracellular reduction of tellurite causes a gunmetal color of the colonies. Center is darker than the periphery. **B.** Blood agar. Colonies are gray and opaque. Unlike staphylococcal colonies, they are dull.

5. C. *diphtheriae* on Löffler's serum. Colonies are small, creamy, granular, and moist.

Plate   8

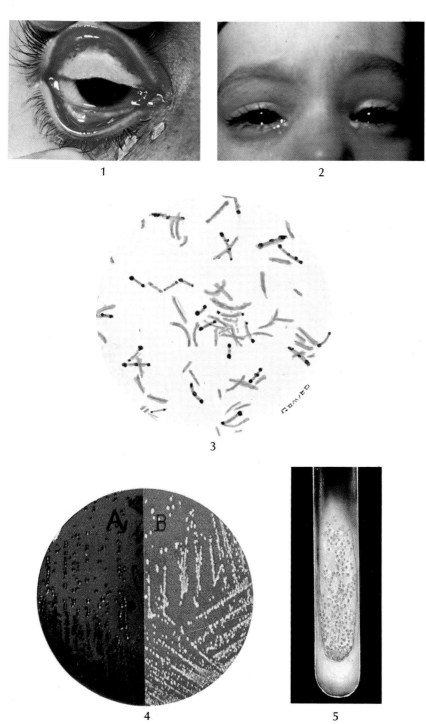

1

2

3

4

5

Plate 9

1. *C. diphtheriae* and *C. xerosis* in smears from culture (Neisser stain). **A.** *C. diphtheriae.* Metachromatic granules are more numerous than in *C. xerosis* and typically located at poles, giving a drumstick appearance. **B.** *C. xerosis.* Metachromatic granules seen in small numbers. Unlike *C. diphtheriae,* these are located throughout the entire organism.

2. In vitro test for virulence. Three streaks show growth of three different strains of corynebacteria. Radiating lines (exaggerated by retouching) seen at streak B indicate that this is the only virulent strain of the three.

3. *C. diphtheriae* and *C. xerosis* cultures. On blood agar: **A.** *C. diphtheriae* colonies are larger than *C. xerosis.* **B.** *C. xerosis* colonies are smaller and drier than *C. diphtheriae.* On Löffler's serum: **C.** *C. diphtheriae* colonies are larger (also faster growing than on blood agar; important for early diagnosis). **D.** *C. xerosis* is smaller and drier than *C. diphtheriae* (growth slower).

4. Fermentation reactions of *C. diphtheriae.* Glucose: positive (yellow). Sucrose: negative (red).

5. *B. subtilis*—gram-positive, aerobic, sporeforming saprophyte. When introduced into the eye, may cause corneal abscess and panophthalmitis. Gram-positive bacilli, except *Corynebacterium* group, are rarely found in eye.

Plate 9

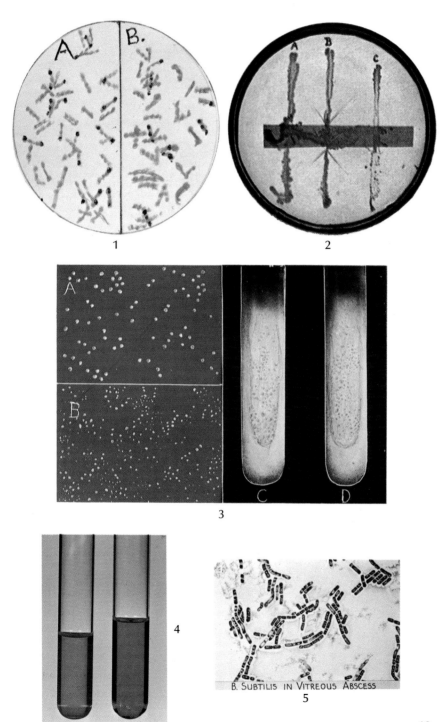

1

2

3

4

5

Plate 10

1. Primary tuberculosis of conjunctiva. Tarsal conjunctiva, which is mainly involved, is much thickened. Conjunctivitis is the papillary type. On top of the papillae, an ulcer often develops, as shown. The condition is associated with oculoglandular Parinaud's syndrome.

2. Deep interstitial keratitis. The keratitis is often in the upper outer quadrant. Vessels penetrate the lesion deeply, in characteristic distribution (unbranched, disappearing at limbus).

3. Unusual, acute, exudative type of ocular tuberculosis. Marked destruction of globe by coalescent necrosis, with resultant cavities. Original smear showed numerous tubercle bacilli. Association with hypersensitivity is assumed.

4. Original smear (Ziehl-Neelsen stain). Acid-fast tubercle bacilli, having granular appearance, arranged predominantly in V forms and resembling corynebacteria.

5. Culture of tubercle bacilli on Löwenstein-Jensen medium (malachite prevents contamination and gives a beautiful green color). Colonies are creamy, dull, rough, and granular. Growth requires at least two months.

Plate 10

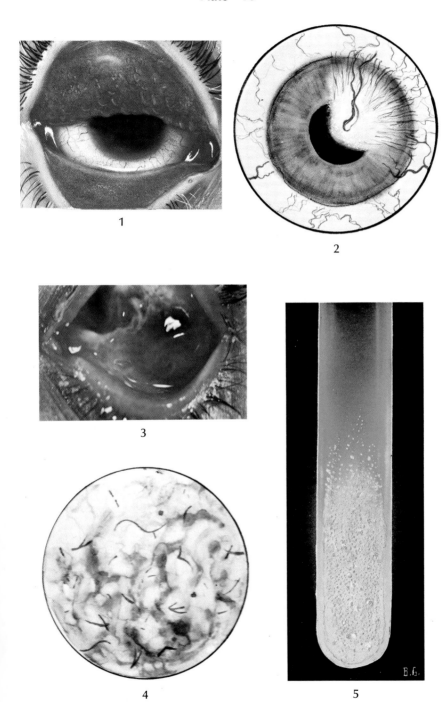

1

2

3

4

5

Plate 11

1. Phlyctenular conjunctivitis **A.** Several small grayish white limbal nodules. Phlyctenules tend to ulcerate. **B.** Solitary nodular phlyctenule.

2. Fascicular keratitis. Note phlyctenule migrating across the cornea, with accompanying vascular tail. (It may extend from limbus to limbus.) The end stage will be a permanent, superficial ribbonlike opacity crossing the cornea.

3. Perforating pustular phlyctenule. Phlyctenules may become acute, purulent, and penetrating. Prolapse of the iris is shown. Perforation then results in adherent leukoma or anterior staphyloma.

4. Eczematous (scrofulous, phlyctenular) pannus. This pannus may involve any or all of the peripheral cornea (trachomatous pannus involves the upper cornea). Superficial vessels beneath the epithelium show arborescent branching.

Plate 11

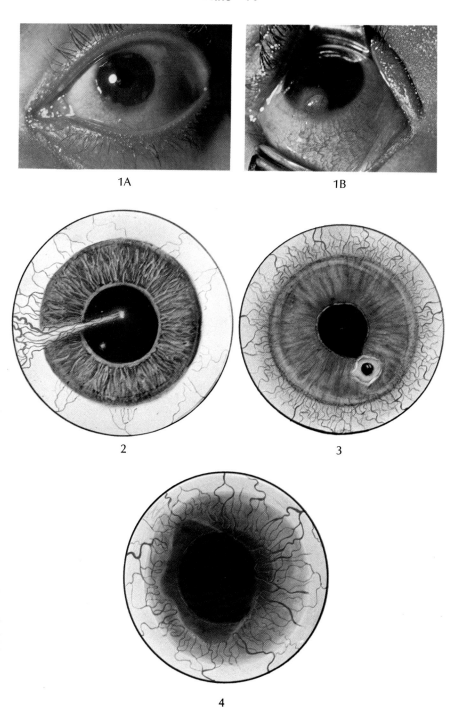

1A

1B

2

3

4

Plate 12

1. Leprotic keratitis. Slit lamp view; small, white opacities and scattered, chalky, minute grains seen in all layers. Note the nodules on the thickened nerves. Hansen's bacilli were found in the corneal scraping. (From patient shown at right.)

2. Nodular leprosy (lepra tuberosa; lepromatous leprosy). Nodules, single or grouped, are typically distributed on the face, mainly on the cheeks, lips, and nose.

3. Multiple, irregular, quiet retinal lesions at the periphery of the fundus. (Same patient as in Fig. 2, above.) The lesions are probably of leprotic origin.

4. Hansen's bacilli in scraping. (From keratitis in Fig. 1, above.) Acid-fast bacilli vary in size and shape. They may be straight, curved, arranged in palisade and V formation, or granular globules. Scraping is sufficient for diagnosis.

5. Corneal leproma. A large, nodular conglomeration (leproma) invading almost the entire cornea. Marked vascularization. The process is asymptomatic and indolent. Many Hansen's bacilli are found in the corneal scraping.

6. Maculoanasthetic leprosy. The process localizes in neuroglia of peripheral nerves, causing lepra claw of the hands. Ocular muscle paresis may occur.

Plate   12

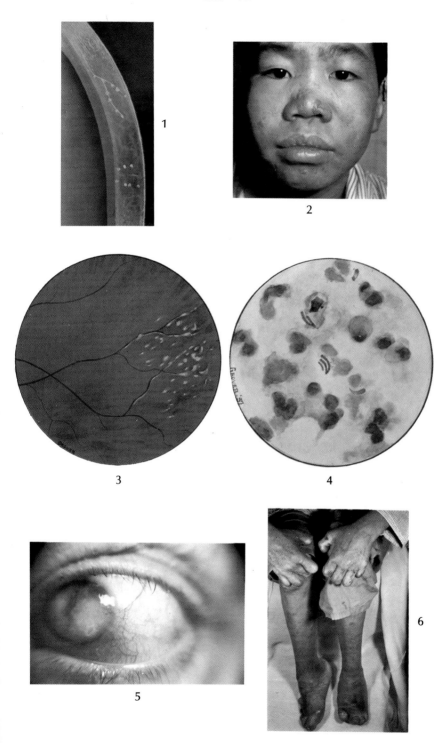

1

2

3

4

5

6

Plate 13

1. Infantile purulent conjunctivitis due to the gonococcus. *N. gonorrhoeae* is the prime offender. Staphylococci, streptococci, or other bacteria may also be causative agents. The conjunctivitis occurs (usually in institutions) in girls aged 2 to 10 by contact with infected sources, human or environmental.

2. Gonococcal ophthalmia neonatorum. General aspect. Note the abundant discharge and marked edema of lids. The examiner should protect his eyes (wearing glasses is best) from spurting pus when he opens the lids.

3. Morphologic characteristics of the gonococcus. **A.** Original smear (gram stain). Smear morphology is more typical than in culture: gram-negative, kidney-shaped diplococci, usually seen within neutrophils. Cell response is mainly neutrophilic. Direct smear is needed, being sufficient for preliminary diagnosis. **B.** Smear from young culture (gram stain). In older culture, gonococci autolyze and die rapidly, showing poorly stained, swollen, and irregular forms.

4. Gonococcal conjunctivitis in adult males, unilateral, characterized by great swelling of lids, copious discharge, and tendency to serious corneal involvement.

5. Gonococci in scraping (Giemsa stain). This shows turflike appearance within and at the edge of epithelial cells. May be found before the exudate smear is positive.

6. Fermentation reactions. Glucose: positive (yellow). Maltose: negative (red).

7. Hyperacute gonococcal conjunctivitis of adult with membrane on upper tarsal conjunctiva.

Plate   13

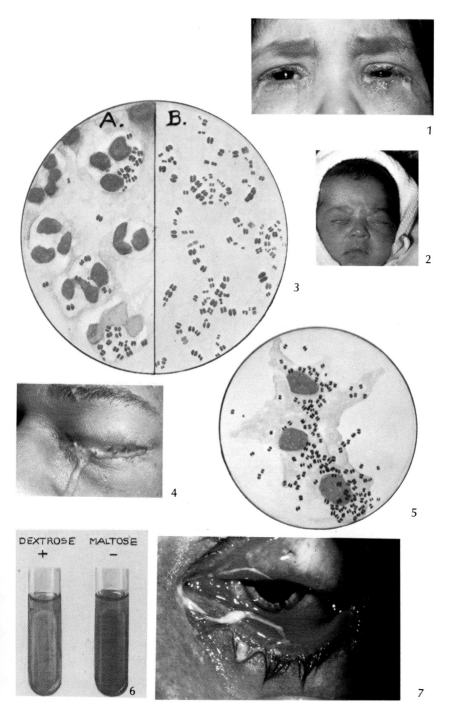

Plate 14

1. Keratitis (slit lamp view). Rare in meningococcal infections. A large area of the cornea is slightly and diffusely opaque, in which area are localized more extensive opacities. One deep vessel is demonstrated in the slit lamp beam.

2. Meningococci in original smear (gram stain). Kidney-shaped, intracellular, diplo-arranged meningococci, morphologically indistinguishable from gonococci.

3. Meningococci in smear from culture (gram stain). Meningococci autolyze and die, not as rapidly as gonococci. Note swollen, poorly stained forms.

4. Fermentation reactions of meningococcus. Maltose: positive (yellow). Glucose: positive (yellow). Sucrose: negative (red).

5. Oxidase test in culture on blood agar. Black spots show a positive oxidase reaction for members of the *Neisseria* genus. By this test, neisseria can be identified in mixed culture.

Plate   14

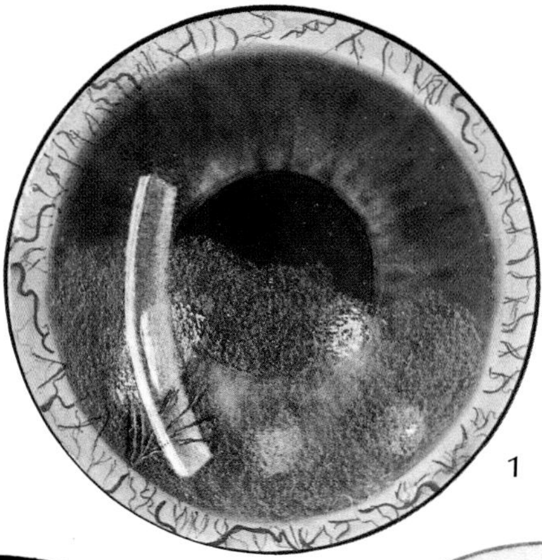

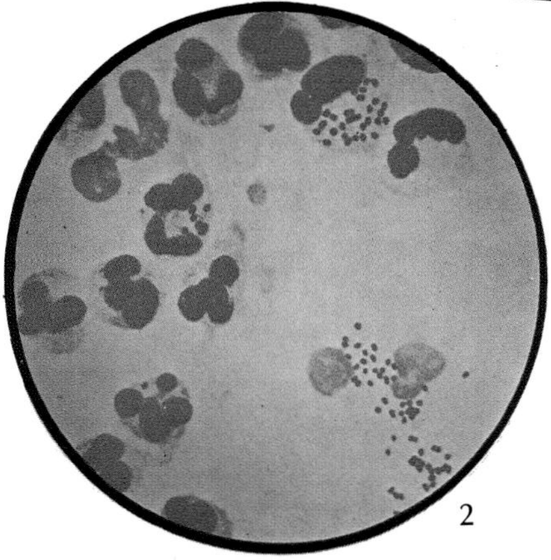

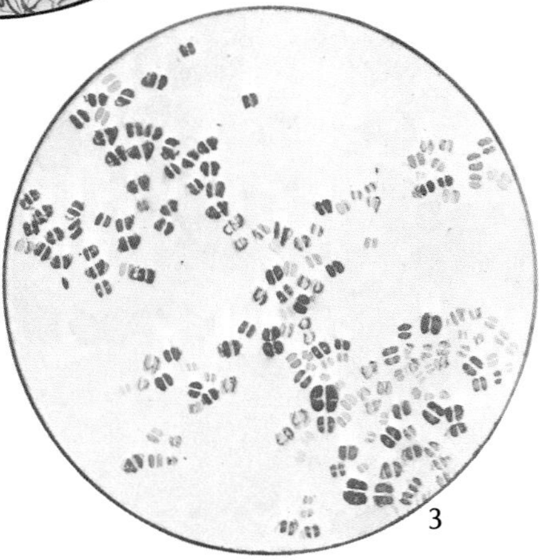

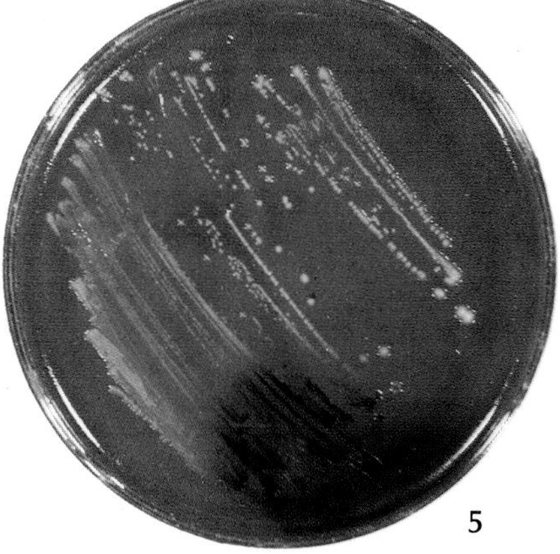

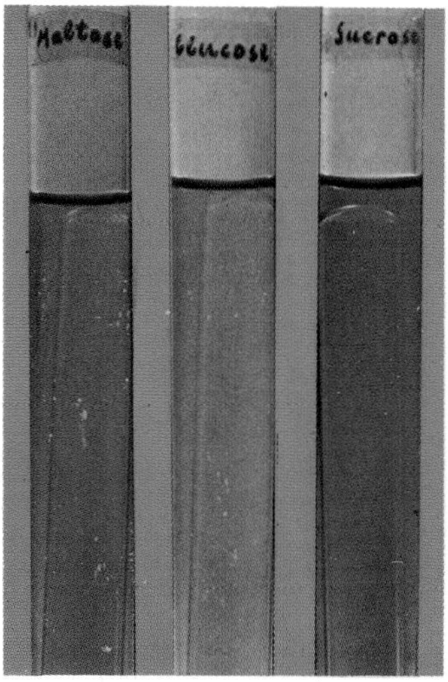

Plate 15

1. *Branchamella catarrhalis (Niesseria)* in original smear (methylene blue stain). Morphology is similar to that of the gonococcus and the meningococcus. Also can be found intracellularly.

2. *Acinetobacter* (Mimeae). Gram-negative cocci found intracellularly. Can be confused with *N. meningitidis* or *N. gonorrhoeae*.

3. *Acinetobacter* in smear from culture. The presence of bacillary forms is the most important differentiation from *Neisseria*, which are cocci.

4. Follicular conjunctivitis associated with prolonged use of mascara. *Acinetobacter* isolated.

5. *B. catarrhalis* culture on plain agar shows good growth. This is the simplest way to distinguish *B. catarrhalis* from the gonococcus and the meningococcus, which do not grow on plain agar.

Plate   15

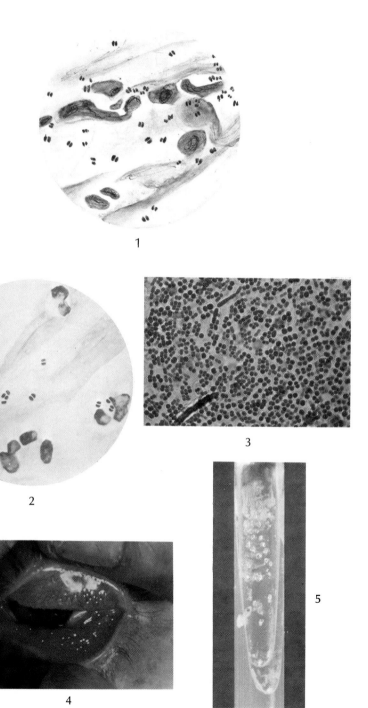

1

2

3

4

5

Plate 16

1. Angular blepharoconjunctivitis due to *M. lacunata*. A chronic process, it may last for years. Numerous diplobacilli are found, even in a mild, asymptomatic process. Without bacteriologic examination, the organism is easily overlooked, and it may complicate intraocular surgery.

2. Central hypopyon keratitis due to *M. lacunata*. Severe, purulent, destructive primary keratitis (without preceding angular blepharoconjunctivitis). This usually appears as a deep abscess and may have intact epithelium in the initial stage. Sterile hypopyon is present, indicating secondary iritis. When the abscess ulcerates, clean out the debris, then scrape the base for bacteriologic diagnosis.

3. Gram-negative diplobacilli in smears (gram stain). **A.** From culture on blood agar. Morphology of the *M. lacunata* usually changes rapidly. Note the pronounced polymorphism from long threads to coccobacilli. Some are club-shaped, resembling corynebacteria. **B.** Original smear from blepharoconjunctivitis exudate. Numerous gram-negative diplobacilli with square-shaped, plump, diplo or short chain appearance (thus distinguishable from other ophthalmic gram-negative bacilli). Also note exudate with many fibrin threads and only a few leukocytes. Direct smear is sufficient for diagnosis. Several *C. xerosis* cells are present, illustrating symbiosis with *M. lacunata*.

4. *M. lacunata* culture on Löffler's serum (grows rapidly). This medium is particularly necessary to demonstrate liquefaction. Note the circumscribed pits (lacunae) typical for *M. lacunata*. No actual colonies of *M. lacunata* are seen. Whitish colonies are *C. xerosis*.

5. Morphology from culture: rapid 24-hour development of huge threads (involution form). Note some fusiform cells.

Plate   16

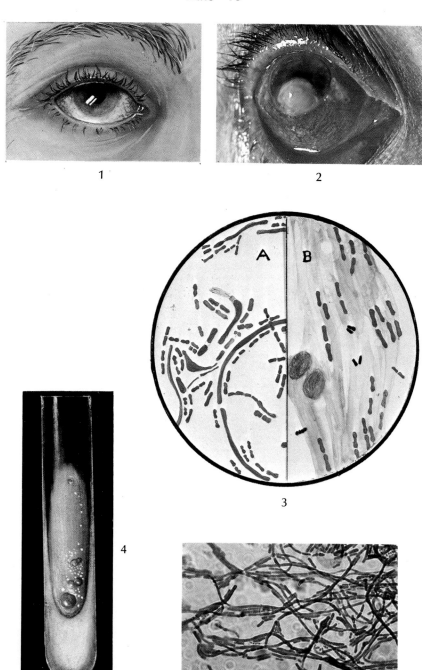

1

2

3

4

5

Plate 17

1. Corneal ulcer with hypopyon due to *M. lacunata* subsp. *liquefaciens,* probably a variant of *M. lacunata.* This is a process similar to that caused by *M. lacunata* (see Plate 16).

2. *M. lacunata* subsp. *liquefaciens* in smear and scraping (gram stain). **A.** From culture on blood agar. Gram-negative diplobacilli. No variation in morphology from that of *M. lacunata.* **B.** Scraping from cornea (same case as Fig. 1, above). Diplobacilli similar to *M. lacunata.* Note a few necrotic corneal epithelial cells.

3. *M. lacunata* subsp. *liquefaciens* culture on Löffler's serum. Liquefaction heavy and confluented. No definite pits (lacunae), as are characteristic for *M. lacunata.*

4. *M. lacunata* subsp. *liquefaciens* culture on blood agar. Diplobacilli grow readily. Colonies are semitransparent and slightly mucoid. No tendency to confluence, no odor.

Plate   17

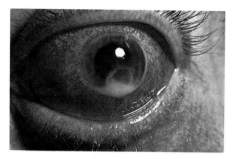

1

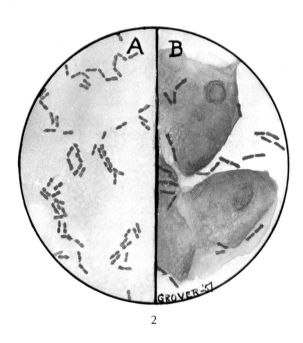

2

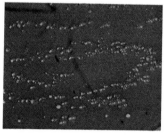

3

4

Plate 18

1. Acute catarrhal conjunctivitis due to the Koch-Weeks bacillus *(H. aegyptius).* Similar to pneumococcal conjunctivitis. Both have intensively hyperemic bulbar conjunctiva and a few petechiae. The discharge is mucopurulent and scanty, with excessive lacrimation. The cornea is rarely involved.

2. Picture demonstrates contagion of the Koch-Weeks bacillus. Family members developed similar acute conjunctivitis within two days.

3. Koch-Weeks bacillus in smears (gram stain). **A.** From culture on blood agar. Gram-negative bacilli are minute, coccobacillary or slender rods. No characteristic arrangement. Often indistinguishable from the enteric group of bacilli. For diagnosis, cultural characteristics are needed. **B.** Original smear of exudate. Slender gram-negative bacilli within leukocytes and between cells are shown. They are difficult to distinguish because of similar background color and minute size.

4. Koch-Weeks bacillus cultures on blood agar and on chocolate agar. **A.** On blood agar. Colonies are tiny, translucent, with a dewdrop appearance. Satellite phenomenon: more luxuriant growth of bacilli around a single staphylococcal colony. **B.** On chocolate agar, colonies are larger than on blood agar. **C.** On blood agar.

5. Candle jar to grow culture in CO_2 atmosphere. The method is simple. Put plates at the bottom of the jar, light the candle, cover the jar. Incubate as usual.

6. Ulcerative keratitis, unusual in *Haemophilus* infection, with diffuse yellowish infiltrate and moderate hypopyon.

Plate   18

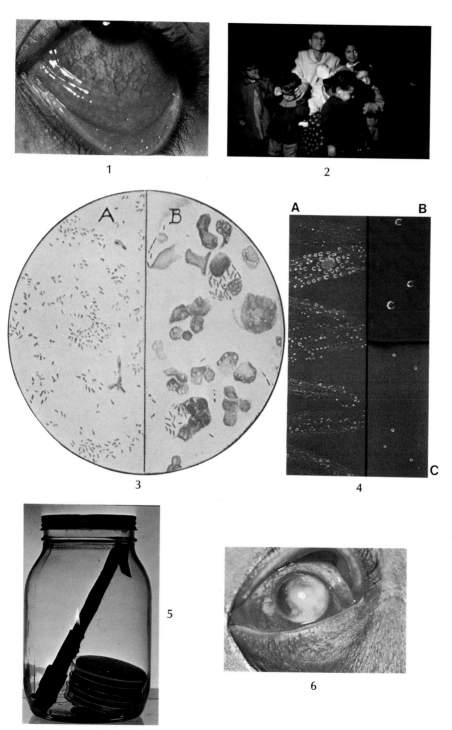

1

2

3

4

5

6

Plate 19

1. *E. coli* and *E. aerogenes*. Smears from culture on blood agar. **A.** *E. coli.* Small, gram-negative bacilli. Pointed or rounded ends stain more intensively (polar stain). Morphologically indistinguishable from other enteric bacilli. Culture is important for diagnosis. **B.** *E. aerogenes*. May be distinguished from other enteric bacilli by its larger size and heavy capsule.

2. *E. coli* culture on MacConkey's agar. Colonies are uniformly pink, large, and dull. This medium is better than blood agar for identification of *E. coli*.

3. Disk sensitivity test for *E. coli*. Single clear zone shows sensitivity of *E. coli* to Kantrex. Sulfonamides, ampicillin, tetracycline, and polymyxins may be markedly effective.

4. Severe, purulent, destructive keratitis due to *E. coli*. Air bubbles can be present in anterior chamber.

5. *E. aerogenes* culture on blood agar. Colonies are easily recognized by their typical heavy, mucoid appearance. No hemolysis.

6. *E. coli* and *E. aerogenes* cultures on EMB agar. *E. coli:* Has characteristic green metallic sheen (left half of plate). *E. aerogenes:* Colonies are dark red in center, colorless on periphery, larger and more mucoid than *E. coli* (right half of plate).

Plate 19

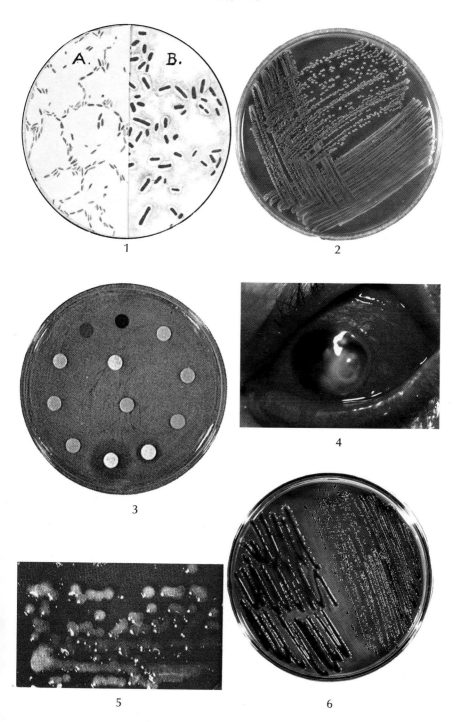

1

2

3

4

5

6

Plate 20

1. Central hypopyon keratitis (caused by nonspreading *Proteus*). A destructive, perforated keratitis, usually associated with trauma. Repeated cultures are necessary, as *P. vulgaris* is often a contaminant.

2. *P. vulgaris* smear from blood agar culture. Small, gram-negative rods with pointed or rounded ends, showing polar stain. Indistinguishable from other gram-negative enteric bacilli.

3. *P. vulgaris* culture on blood agar. Note swarming growth over entire plate. The scratch crossing the circular waves was made to emphasize the diffuse, filmy growth. These waves indicate periodic growth. A putrid odor is detected at a distance.

4. Tests for differentiation of the enteric group. Russell double sugar agar (left tube): indicates lactose-negative (butt is acid, slant is alkaline). Simmon's citrate agar slant (middle tube): indicates citrate-negative. SIM medium (right tube): indicates indol-positive and H_2S-positive.

5. *Serratia bacillus*, producing red pigment. Culture on plain agar.

6. DNAase reaction indicates virulence of *S. marcescens*. Note light zone around culture (other nonpathogens show negative reaction).

Plate   20

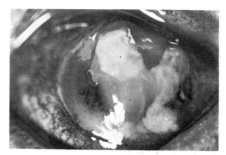

1

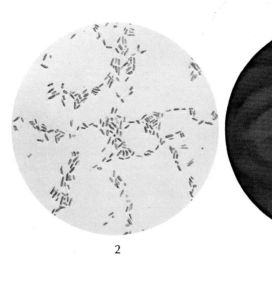

2

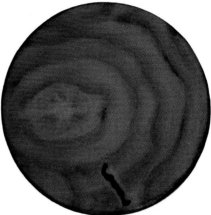

3

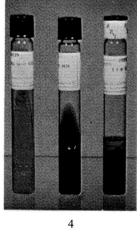

4

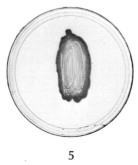

5

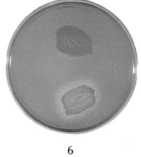

6

Plate 21

1. *P. aeruginosa* smear from culture (gram stain). Small gram-negative rods (as are other enteric bacilli). Culture is necessary for diagnosis.

2. *P. aeruginosa* culture on blood agar. Colonies and surrounding medium are a dark greenish gray due to pigment production. The strong, sweet odor is an important diagnostic aid.

3. Central hypopyon keratitis due to *P. aeruginosa*. The process is characterized by severe and rapid necrosis, often resulting in perforation and panophthalmitis. Laboratory diagnosis followed by intensive therapy is urgent.

4. Bilateral lacrimal mucocele. This condition results from prolonged chronic dacryocystitis; an atonic sac with exudate is present. Mixed flora is usually found. This case was unusual, as a pure culture of *P. aeruginosa* was isolated.

5. Fluorescein solution. *P. aeruginosa* contaminates fluorescein solution readily, presenting a serious ophthalmologic problem.

6. Disk sensitivity test for *P. aeruginosa*. Sensitivity indicated by two zones of inhibition (the larger, polymyxin B; the narrower, streptomycin). Gentamycin, carbenicillin, or chloramphenicol may be most successful if treatment is begun early.

Plate 21

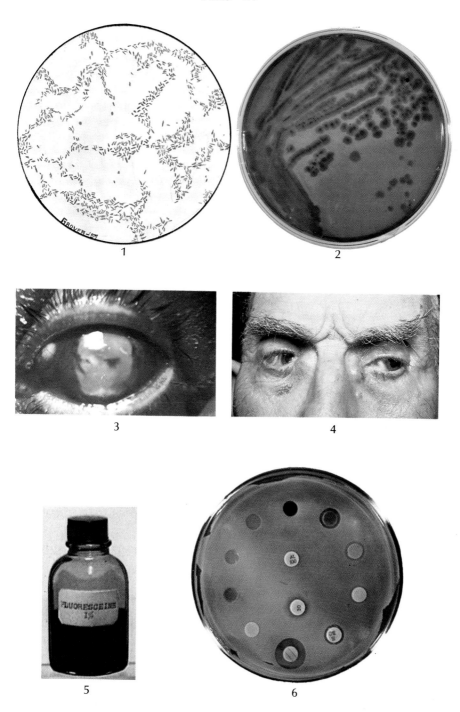

1

2

3

4

5

6

Plate 22

1. Cytology of trachoma in scraping (Giemsa stain). Note basophilic cytoplasmic inclusion bodies (Prowazek) in epithelial cells. Lymphocytes and plasma cells are typically found in trachoma.

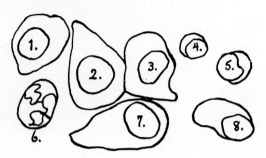

1.		4.	
2.	Basophilic cytoplasmic inclusion	5.	Lymphocytes
3.	bodies (Prowazek) in epithelial	6.	Neutrophil
7.	cells	8.	Plasma cell

2. Cytoplasmic granules. These are not to be confused with trachomatous inclusion bodies.

3. Pathology of trachoma in section (hematoxylin-eosin stain). Follicles are shown, each consisting of a peripheral zone of lymphocytes and a germinal center of large lymphoblasts, monocytes, and epithelioid cells. Note round cell infiltration of stroma. On the right, a hypertrophic papilla with beginning fibrosis (red streaks) is shown.

4. Leber cell. The Leber cell is a giant macrophage, significant but not specific for trachoma. Its cytoplasmic border is ill-defined. The cytoplasm engulfs debris from disintegrated cells (nuclear material is dark, cytoplasmic is light).

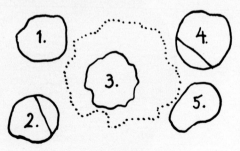

1.		
2.	Degenerated lymphocytes	3. Leber cell
4.		
5.		

Plate 22

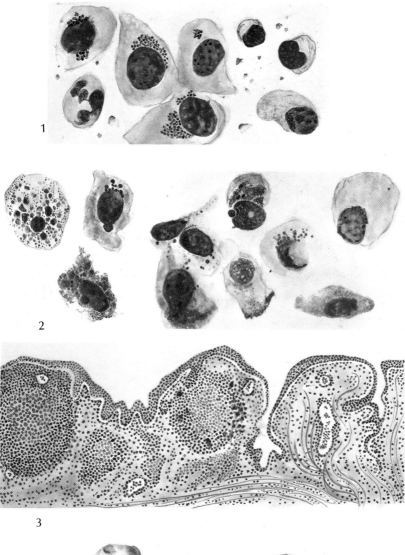

1

2

3

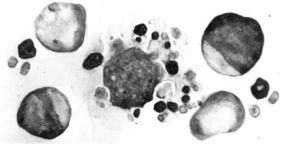

4

Plate 23

1. Pannus trachomatosus. Diffuse vascular keratitis. Typically, the superficial branching vessels invade the upper limbus and run subepithelially in the cornea. Note the diffuse opacity and two isolated infiltrates.

2. Trachomatous follicular conjunctivitis in the early stage of trachoma. The follicles are indistinguishable from those in other follicular conjunctivitis or folliculosis. Localization on upper tarsal conjunctiva, with infiltration of surrounding tissue, is significant for differential diagnosis of early trachoma.

3. Scarring of upper tarsal conjunctiva in trachoma. The scar is usually horizontal, particularly along the sulcus subtarsalis; entropion often results.

4. Trachomatous ptosis. The upper lid droops due to the weight of the infiltrated lid or from infiltration of the levator muscle at the site of its insertion.

5. Consequences of trachoma: total corneal scarring, trichiasis, pseudopterygium.

Plate 23

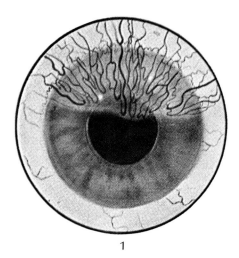

1

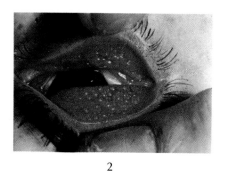

2

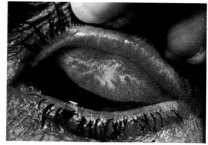

3

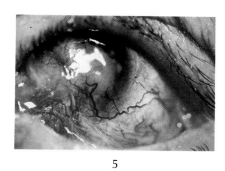

4

5

Plate 24

1. Inclusion conjunctivitis of newborn. Acute purulent conjunctivitis occuring 5 to 10 days after birth. Conjunctiva of lower lid is predominantly involved; take the scraping from the lower conjunctiva. The process is usually mild. In severe cases pseudomembranes occur. The cornea is uninvolved. Cytoplasmic basophilic inclusion bodies (illustrated in Fig. 3) confirm the diagnosis.

2. Inclusion conjunctivitis of adults, undistinguishable from viral. Process may begin as an unilateral acute bacterial conjunctivitis (moderate secretion). Later the other eye is usually involved and follicles appear; papillary hypertrophy may develop.

3. Scraping (Giemsa stain) from inclusion conjunctivitis. Cytoplasmic basophilic inclusion bodies in epithelial cells are indistinguishable from those in trachoma. In the typical cell response, neutrophils and monocytes are seen. Monocytes are usually vacuolized. Giant multinucleated cells may be found.

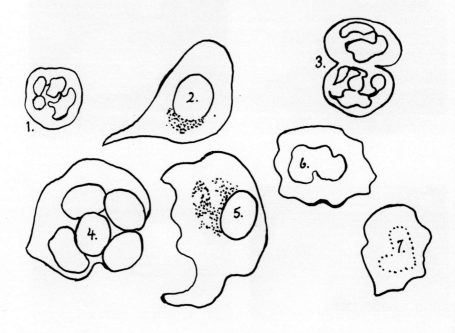

1. ⎱
3. ⎰ Neutrophils

4.   Multinucleated cell

2. ⎱ Epithelial cells with Prowazek's
5. ⎰ inclusion bodies

6. ⎱ Monocytes with vacuolization
7. ⎰ and autolysis

48

Plate   24

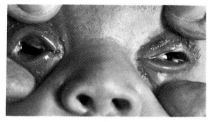

1

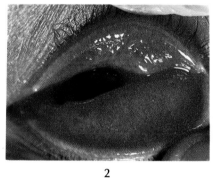

2

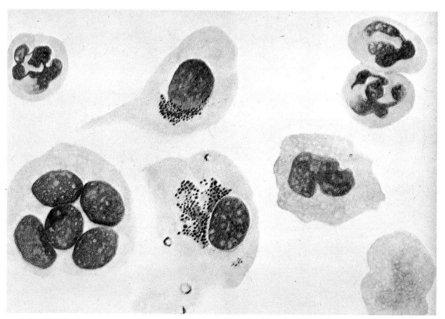

3

Plate 25

1. Sequelae of corneal variola pustule. Anterior staphyloma, with resulting permanent blindness. Note pox marks on skin.

2. Vaccinial disciform keratitis (similar to other disciform keratitis). A type of avascular interstitial keratitis. The opacity is not dense. The process is benign. Grayish lines near the disk are Descemet's folds.

3. Vaccinia of lid. Typical transmission to lid (inner angulus usual) from the site of vaccination, showing on arm.

4. Guarnieri variola-vaccinia inclusion bodies (Giemsa stain). Inclusions are eosinophilic, cytoplasmic (in variola, intranuclear as well), consisting of Paschen's elementary bodies. Guarnieri bodies are rarely found except in experimental studies. Ballooning degeneration, monocytes, and neutrophils are additional cytologic characteristics.

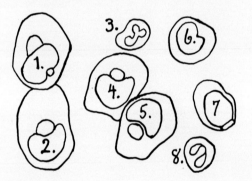

1.
2. } Cytoplasmic eosinophilic
4. } Guarniery inclusion bodies
5.

6. Monocyte

3.
8. } Neutrophils

7. Ballooning degeneration

50

Plate 25

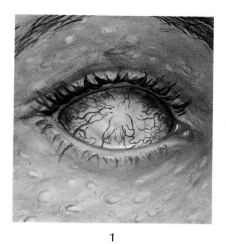

1

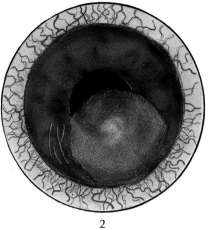

2

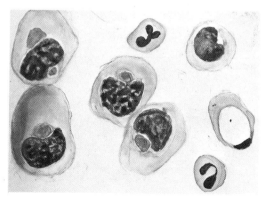

3

4

Plate 26

1. Zoster (herpes zoster, shingles, zona). Severe ulcerative necrotic process distributed along supraorbital branch. Usually unilateral (except in syphilis).

2. Disciform keratitis (usual type). The corneal disk-shaped opacity in the interstitial tissue is not dense; its surface may be eroded. Descemet's folds sometimes occur.

3. Dendritic keratitis in zoster (typically peripheral).

4. Cytology in scraping (Giemsa stain). Eosinophilic, intranuclear Lipschütz inclusion bodies (similar to those in *H. simplex)* are pictured. Ballooning degeneration and multinucleated giant cells are additional findings.

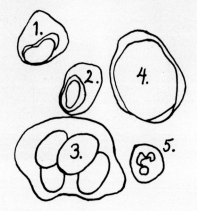

1. } Eosinophilic intranuclear
2. } Lipschütz inclusion bodies

3.   Multinucleated giant cell

5.   Neutrophil

4.   Ballooning degeneration

5. Varicella. Although a disease of childhood, varicella virus may become latent and manifest as a zoster in adulthood.

Plate 26

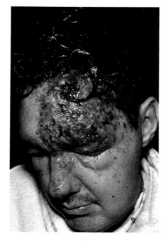

1

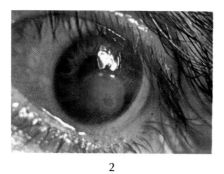

2

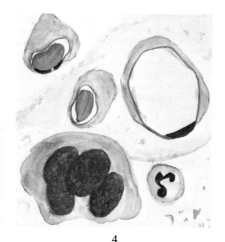

3

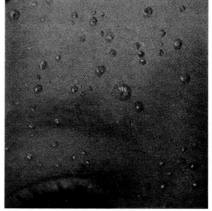

4

5

Plate 27

1. Primary bilateral dendritic corneal ulcers in newborn baby. This condition is rare, usually bilateral, and accompanied by systemic manifestations. Dendritic shape and loss of sensitivity indicate herpetic origin.

2. Recurrent dendritic corneal ulcer (in adult). Commonly chronic, unilateral, and recurrent. Branching figure and loss of corneal sensitivity are regarded as pathognomonic for *H. simplex*. No systemic manifestations. (Slit lamp picture.)

3. Cytology in scraping (Giemsa stain). Eosinophilic intranuclear Lipschütz inclusion bodies similar to zoster. Giant multinucleated cell, usually found in *H. simplex* infection. Monocytes and neutrophils are commonly found.

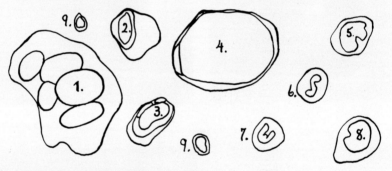

1. Giant multinucleated cell	5. ⎱ Monocytes 8. ⎰
2. ⎱ Eosinophilic intranuclear 3. ⎰ Lipschütz inclusion bodies	6. ⎱ Neutrophils 7. ⎰
4. Cell showing ballooning degeneration	9. Debris

4. Giant multinucleated cell (in scraping)—significant for *H. simplex*.

5. Variety of multinucleated giant cells in *H. simplex* infection.

6. Disciform keratitis (late stage). Dense, deep opacity invaded by deep vessels; scarring results.

7. Old dendritic keratitis, no inflammatory reaction.

Plate   27

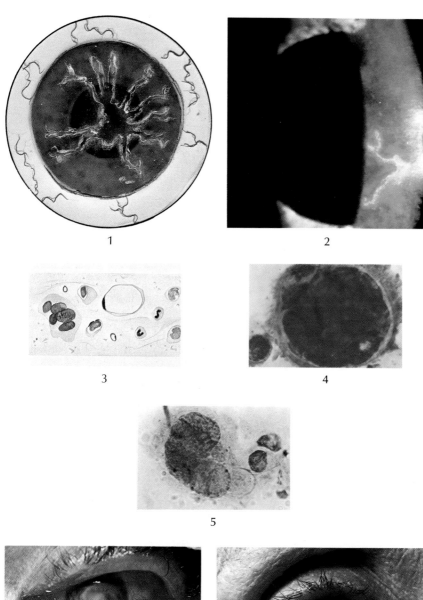

1   2

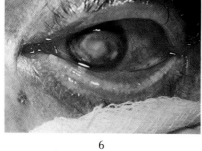

3   4

5

6   7

Plate 28

1. Acute herpetic blepharitis. Several broken vesicles are present on the margin and skin of the lids. The lids are markedly swollen. Preauricular glands are enlarged.

2. Acute herpetic follicular conjunctivitis. Lower conjunctiva is involved. Note a few skin vesicles at inner angle.

3. Acute herpetic blepharoconjunctivitis. Along the cilial line broken vesicles have resulted in an ulcerated area which, unlike usual blepharitis, is covered by a grayish membrane. Follicular conjunctivitis, mainly in the lower fornix, developed two days after onset. Enlargement of preauricular and submaxillary glands.

4. Follicular conjunctivitis associated with mild sore throat and fever (pharyngoconjunctival fever). Follicles are localized mainly in the lower fornix, and inner angle. Enlargment of preauricular and, particularly, submaxillary glands. Adenovirus type 3 was isolated.

5. Epidemic keratoconjunctivitis (EKC). Subepithelial, small, grayish, irregular, multiple lesions. Localization in central (pupillary) area is typical for EKC. The disease was evidently caused by adenovirus type 8.

6. Cytology in scraping (Giemsa stain). Mononuclear cells: monocytes and lymphocytes predominate. Large epithelial cells may be found. Similar cytology is found in other viral conjunctivitides.

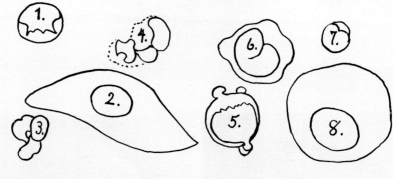

1.
5. } Lymphocytes
7.

3. } Neutrophils
4.

6. Monocyte

2. } Large epithelial cells
8.

Plate 28

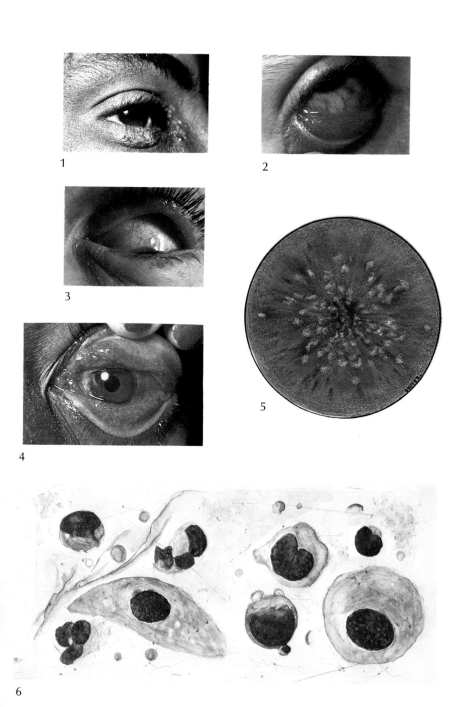

1

2

3

5

4

6

Plate 29

1. Molluscum contagiosum of lids. Uninflamed, round, waxy, white lesion at lid margin. The summit is usually umbilicated and has a tiny black spot. If the lesion is situated at the lid margin, the cornea and conjunctiva can be involved.

2. Follicular conjunctivitis due to molluscum contagiosum. Note lesion on upper lid margin.

3. Pannus develops if molluscum lesion is situated at the lid margin. This is localized (similarly to trachoma) at the upper part of the cornea. Probably toxic in origin, it heals after removal of lid lesion. It is usually associated with chronic follicular conjunctivitis.

4. Inclusion bodies of molluscum contagiosum (in section, stained with hematoxylin-eosin). Henderson-Paterson cytoplasmic eosinophilic inclusion bodies. These are composed of elementary bodies aggregated in globular masses (separated by septa) which press the shrunken nucleus (shown by dark staining) to the cell wall.

5. Cornu cutaneum (cutaneous horn). A rare lesion consisting of horny epithelium; regarded as horn wart, probably viral.

6. Warts (verruca filiformis). Epidermal and papillary growths of viral origin; soft and flexible, typically situated on face, neck, and eyelids. Multiple lesions are disseminated in the bearded area by shaving. Involvement of the cornea and conjunctiva (as in molluscum contagiosum) may occur if the lesion is situated at the lid margin.

Plate 29

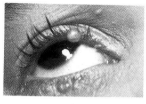

1

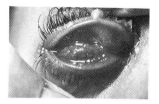

2

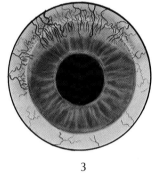

3

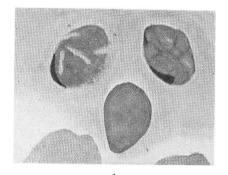

4

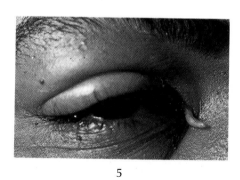

5

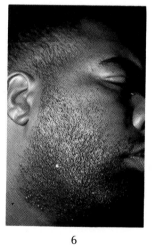

6

Plate 30

1. Mycotic canaliculitis shown in upper canaliculus. The surrounding area is swollen but not inflamed. White spot is an exudate. Dilatation of punctum and chronic, unilateral conjunctivitis aid diagnosis. *Streptothrix*, the usual causative organism, is anaerobic, making cultivation difficult, and the process is often overrun by bacteria. Direct smear is used for preliminary diagnosis. Actinomycetes are susceptible to antibacterial but not to antifungal agents.

2. Diverticulum of lower canaliculus found in long-lasting canaliculitis.

3. *Nocardia* grows aerobically and slowly (three to four weeks) on Sabouraud's medium. Colonies are wrinkled, crumbling, and resemble mycobacteria (blood agar culture).

4. Exudate smear from canaliculitis—branched and unbranched filaments of streptothrix. Fragments readily into bacillary and coccal elements, confused with bacteria commonly found. Examination of smear is essential for diagnosis, and culture is difficult.

5. *Leptothrix:* smear from film on teeth. Long, unbranched filaments are typical for saprophytic strain. (Found in Parinaud's syndrome.)

Plate   30

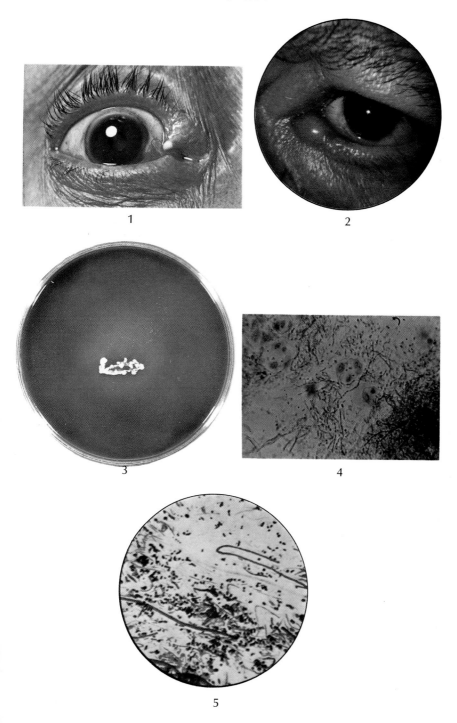

1

2

3

4

5

Plate 31

1. Mycotic keratitis due to *C. albicans* (from a case of generalized, fatal candidiasis). Multiple elevated corneal lesions, yellowish and definitely marginated. The process is indolent, with moderate inflammation. Also note multiple, isolated, quiet skin lesions. Diagnosis is confirmed by laboratory studies.

2. Hypopyon keratitis. *C. albicans* isolated. The abscesslike keratitis is ulcerated in the center and covered by a brownish, necrotic mass resembling bread crumbs. *C. albicans* found in corneal scraping.

3. Thrush. Develops after prolonged use of antibiotics. Other lesions on the skin, including the eyelid, are definitely marginated, accompanied by blepharitis and dermatitis.

4. *C. albicans* in original corneal scraping (gram stain). Yeastlike bodies of *C. albicans* and pseudomycelia are illustrated.

5. Endophthalmitis due to *C. albicans*, in drug addict. (Courtesy of Dr. M. Spinack, Montefiore Hospital Medical Center.)

Plate 31

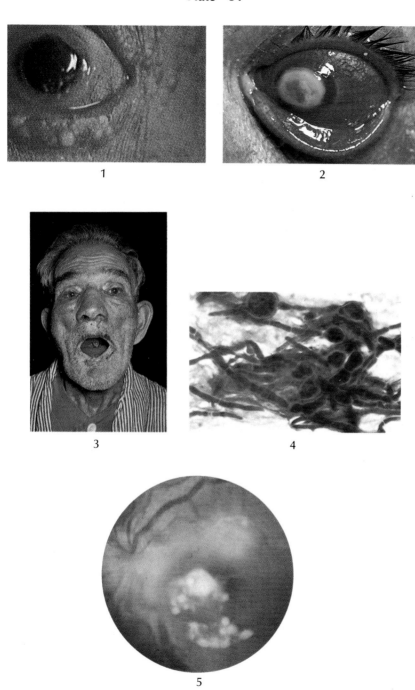

1

2

3

4

5

Plate 32

1. *C. albicans* in smear from culture on blood agar (gram stain). Gram-positive, round bodies in cluster arrangement can be distinguished from staphylococci by their larger size, budding, and more intense gram stain.

2. Chlamydospores from cornmeal medium; a few mycelia are present (cotton blue mount). (Courtesy of Dr. S. A. Rosenthal, New York University.)

3. *C. albicans* culture on Sabouraud's medium: colonies are small, round, opaque, dry or moist, as are staphylococcal colonies. They have a yeastlike odor and morphology.

4. Germ tube technique important for diagnosis of *C. albicans*. Inoculate 1 ml of fetal calf serum with organisms from the culture, incubate two to three hours at 37 C, and examine microscopically. (Courtesy of Dr. S. A. Rosenthal, New York University.)

Plate 32

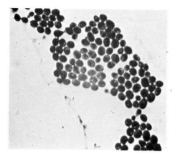

1

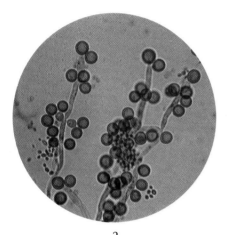

2

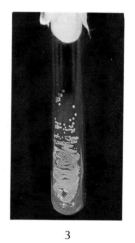

3

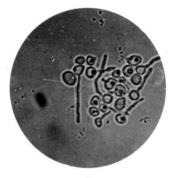

4

Plate 33

1. Choked disk. Papilledema has occasionally been associated with systemic blastomycosis.

2. *B. dermatitidis* on Sabouraud's medium. White, cottony colonies later become brownish and prickly, as in center. Growth requires four weeks or more.

3. *B. dermatitidis* in tissue, PAS stain. Budding, double-contoured yeastlike cells typical for this fungus are seen. (Courtesy of Dr. S. A. Rosenthal, New York University.)

4. *H. capsulatum*, mycelial phase. Smear from Sabouraud's culture (cotton blue mount). (Courtesy of Dr. S. A. Rosenthal, New York University.)

5. *H. capsulatum* is shown within mononuclear cell in biopsy specimen. The oval yeastlike bodies resemble protozoa. (Courtesy of Dr. S. A. Rosenthal, New York University.)

6. *H. capsulatum* on Sabouraud's medium. Colonies are cottony white, becoming brown in old culture. Growth requires at least three weeks.

7. *H. capsulatum* subculture on blood agar.

8. *H. duboisii* in tissue, full of encapsulated forms (PAS stain). (Courtesy of Dr. S. A. Rosenthal, New York University.)

Plate 33

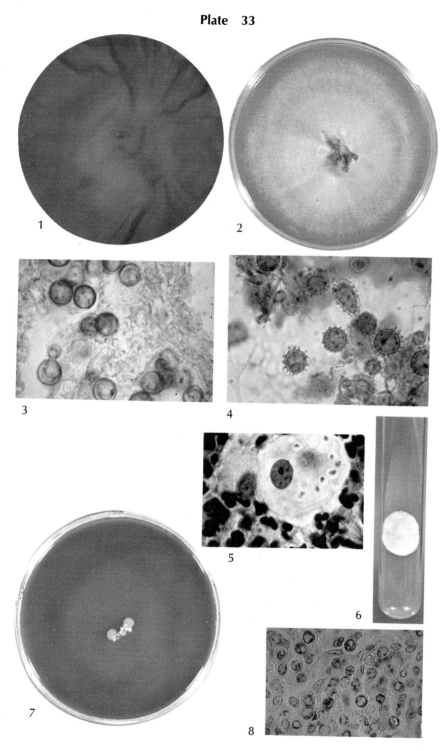

Plate 34

1. Granulomatous skin ulcer caused by *C. neoformans*. Such local lesions may lead to systemic infection. Cryptococcosis may coexist with other diseases (Hodgkin's disease, sarcoid), creating a bizarre clinical picture.

2. Chorioretinitis, exudate in vitreus. *C. neoformans* was found in culture. (Courtesy of Dr. M. Spinack, Montefiore Hospital Medical Center.)

3. *C. neoformans* (India ink preparation). This staining method demonstrates the thick walls of the yeastlike cells, important for identification. Some cells show budding.

4. *C. neoformans* in tissue (GE stain). Thick-walled cells shown. (Courtesy of Dr. S. A. Rosenthal, New York University.)

5. Spherule of *Coccidioides immitis*. Contains numerous round or oval spores—differentiation from blastomyces. External and internal eye can be involved.

6. *C. neoformans* in smear from blood agar culture (Giemsa stain). Polygonal bodies, with honeycomblike arrangement.

7. *C. neoformans* on Sabouraud's medium. Colonies are mucoid and slimy, resembling cultures of Friedländer's bacillus.

Plate 34

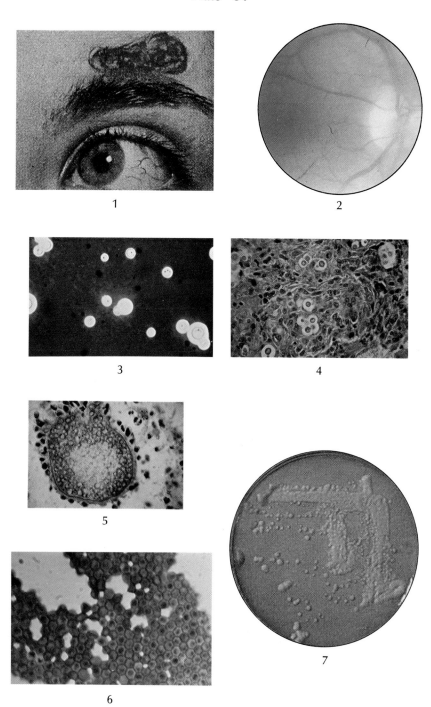

1

2

3

4

5

6

7

Plate 35

1. *Fusarium* fungal corneal ulcer, showing raised whitish lesion with hyphate edges. (Courtesy of Dr. H. J. Kaufman, Gainesville, Florida.)

2. *Fusarium* fungal dry-looking, painful keratitis at beginning stage. Several slightly grayish spots in superficial corneal layers. No hypopyon, no marked inflammatory reaction.

3. Corneal scraping from patient shown in Fig. 2. The occasional septated mycelium was found in gram-stained preparation.

4. Morphology of *Fusarium* in smear from culture (blue cotton mount). Septate spindle hyphae are demonstrated. (Courtesy of Dr. S. A. Rosenthal, New York University.)

5. Culture of *Fusarium*. (Courtesy of Dr. S. A. Rosenthal, New York University.)

6. *Curvularia* species keratitis showing raised whitish lesion with hyphate edges. (Courtesy of Dr. H. J. Kaufman, Gainesville, Florida.)

7. Raised whitish lesion with endothelial plaque and hypopyon. (Courtesy of Dr. H. J. Kaufman, Gainesville, Florida.)

Plate 35

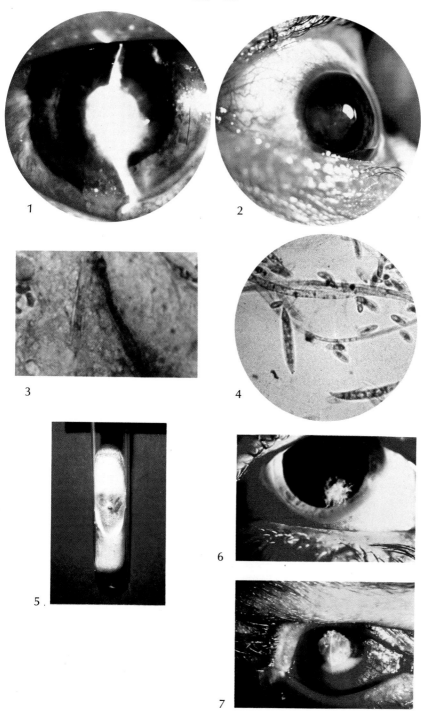

Plate 36

1. Seborrheic blepharitis (sicca). Lashes and brows are heavily powdered with scales—so-called dandruff of lids. Scalp dandruff is always present. *P. ovale* is invariably found. The condition is frequently aggravated by staphylococcal infection.

2. *P. ovale* in scraping from lid margin (methylene blue stain). Ophthalmic *P. ovale* is predominantly round, while scalp *P. ovale* is flask-shaped. When staining, wash the preparation carefully, as greasy secretion slips off easily. Cultivation is difficult, and scraping suffices for diagnosis.

3. *P. ovale* in smear from culture (Giemsa stain). Spherical forms predominate. *P. ovale* differs from staphylococci in being larger, taking a lighter stain in center, and having budding cells.

4. *P. ovale* culture (Littman's agar plate with olive oil). Seborrheic scales from lid are seeded on plate. Confluented colonies swimming on oil have an oily appearance; otherwise they are similar to many yeasts. Growth takes about seven days.

5. *P. ovale* culture on Sabouraud's medium (with olive oil). Growth is slower than on Littman's agar. Colonies are gray, opaque, and often confluented.

Plate 36

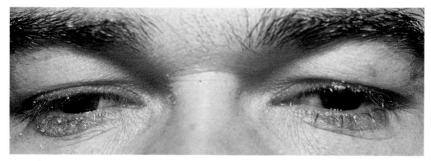

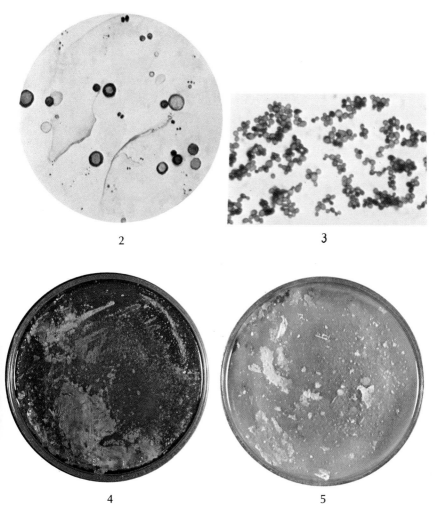

1

2

3

4

5

Plate 37

1. *Penicillium* species culture on Sabouraud's medium. Grows readily. Colonies are white, later become bluish green and powdery. *Penicillium* is a common culture contaminant, occasionally pathogenic. It is rare in eye pathology. It has been recorded as a secondary invader in streptococcal infection of corneal transplant after heavy treatment with antibiotics.

2. Sporebearing hyphae of *Penicillium*. Hyphae, in the form of a brush, have abundant conidia (spores at ends of conidiophores). This structure identifies *Penicillium*. (Courtesy of Dr. S. A. Rosenthal, New York University.)

3. *A. niger* in culture on Sabouraud's medium. This is the commonest culture contaminant. Occasionally it causes granulomatous infection (sinus, external ear, lung, eye). In the eye, aspergillosis of the inferior canaliculus, with molasseslike discharge, occurs rarely. Aspergillus may cause granuloma of the orbit (secondary to sinusitis) or hypopyon keratitis (following injury). In both, a molasseslike discharge may be seen. It is difficult to determine the etiologic role of *Aspergillus*.

4. Sporebearing hyphae of *Aspergillus*. Conidiabearing, unbranched, nonseptate hyphae are needed for identification of Aspergillus.

5. Fungi commonly found as laboratory contaminants. Those pictured include *Aspergillus, Penicillium, Mucor,* and unidentified fungi. *Mucor* can be an ocular pathogen, usually seen in diabetes. The systemic mycosis is frequently fatal.

Plate   37

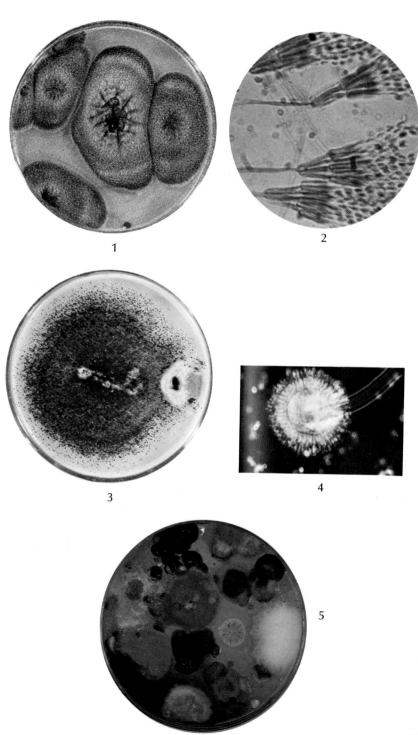

1

2

3

4

5

Plate 38

1. Palpebral vernal conjunctivitis (spring catarrh). Marked hypertrophy of papillae, which are hard and flattened. Vascularization of papillae is reticular, resembling petechiae (with slit lamp). Cobblestone and milky appearance differentiates the condition from trachoma. The fornix is not affected. Eosinophils are commonly found.

2. Fibrosis of upper tarsal conjunctiva, consequence of spring catarrh. Results from prolonged process, or overtreatment (particularly with antibiotics) when wrongly diagnosed. Pathologic features: fibrosis, hyaline degeneration, and eosinophilic infiltration.

3. Vernal conjunctivitis, limbal type. Several grayish, limbal lesions of milky appearance, with tendency to confluence. Distinguished from phlyctenules by absence of vascularization and ulceration. Scraping reveals eosinophils. The condition is often associated with Togby's keratitis (epithelialis vernalis), which has a dusty, flourlike appearance.

4. Vernal conjunctivitis of long duration, shows marked hyaline degeneration. Cornea involved, interstitial keratitis typically in center, resembling sclerosing type.

5. Cytology in scraping from vernal conjunctivitis (Giemsa stain).

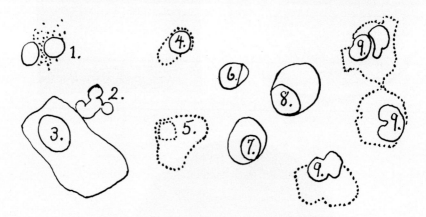

1.
4. Eosinophils in various
5. stages of development
9.

7. Plasma cells
8.

6. Lymphocyte

3. Epithelial cell

2. Segmented nucleus of leukocyte, with cytoplasmic autolysis

Plate 38

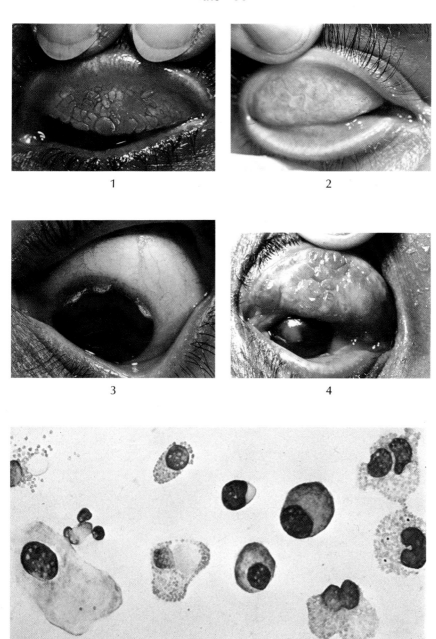

1

2

3

4

5

Plate 39

1. Mouse bite: **A.** Bitten area of external angulus. **B.** Marginal keratitis extended from indurated yellowish white ulcerated lesion at limbus. Marked hyperemia, moderate chemosis shown. Recovery after one week.

2. Pediculosis palpebrarum **A.** Head louse with nits attached to hair. Blepharitis sometimes associated with follicular conjunctivitis. **B.** *Phtirius pubis.*

3. Nodular acute unilateral conjunctivitis. Note the distinct round nodules topped by a yellow spot. The bulbar conjunctiva is also involved. Preauricular and submaxillary glands are enlarged. Laboratory tests for bacterial and fungal infections, including *Leptothrix* (in section), were negative. Conjunctival scraping showed eosinophils; the patient's white blood count revealed 10 percent eosinophilia. An unusual allergic reaction was suggested.

4. Sensitivity reaction to atropine. This may develop after a single instillation.

5. Atopic dermatitis. Shows pustular and exfoliated stage.

6. Cytology in conjunctival scraping (from acute conjunctivitis of toxic or allergic origin).

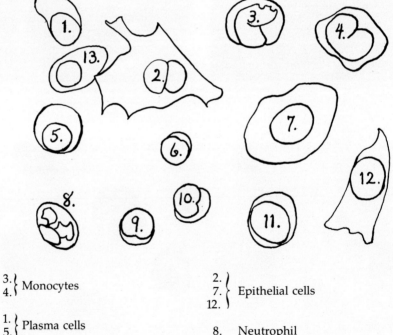

3.
4. } Monocytes

1.
5. } Plasma cells

6.
9.
10.
11. } Lymphocytes

2.
7. } Epithelial cells
12.

8.   Neutrophil

13.   Mast cell

Plate 39

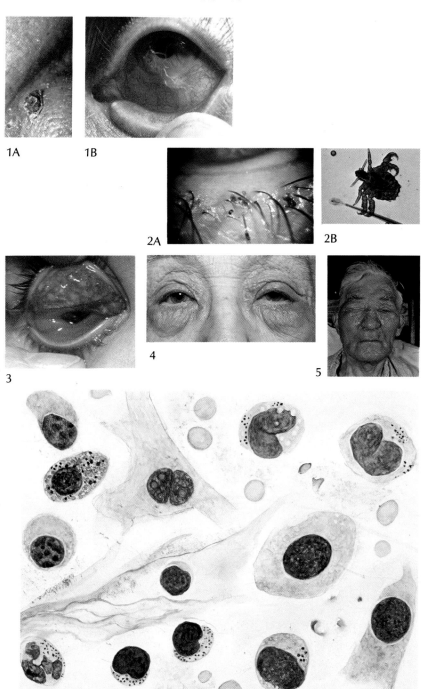

1A

1B

2A

2B

3

4

5

6

Plate 40

1. Epithelial erosion, keratitis sicca, varies from a few erosions to severest destructive changes. Dry epithelium may develop rapidly as a sign of toxicity, IDU (idoxuridine) and other drugs, particularly in the aged.

2. Keratitis sicca in female with Jogren's syndrome. Recurrent dramatic necrosis of cornea with sequestrated area. This was ulcerated and perforated. The same picture recurred on the corneal graft.

3. Essential shrinkage at late stage, fornix almost completely obliterated by fibrosed tissue. Deep complete corneal scarring with granulomalike vascularization.

4. Acute membranous conjunctivitis (early stage) in Stevens-Johnson disease. Probably of toxic origin.

5. Degenerated cornea in late stage of Stevens-Johnson disease. The surface is dry, rough and keratinized—xerophthalmia.

Plate 40

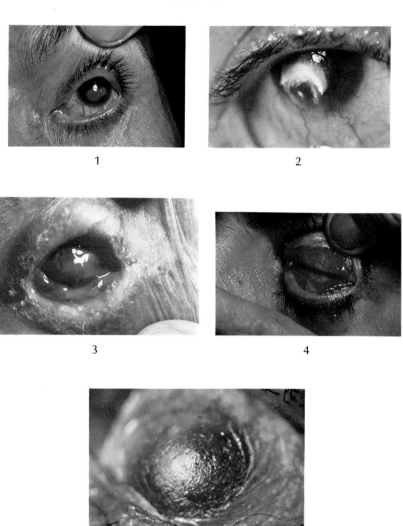

1

2

3

4

5

Plate 41

1. Corneal dermoid (very rarely occurs). The corneal tissue replaced by fibrofatty yellow growth. Epidermal structures, such as hair follicles and sebaceous and sweat glands, are usually present.

2. Folliculosis (adenitis of conjunctiva: Duke-Elder). Abundant, large, discrete, semitransparent, pinkish yellow follicles. They are arranged in rows, mainly in the lower fornix, and are not found on bulbar conjunctiva. Lack of inflammation and absence of trachomatous inclusion bodies are important for differentiation. It is mainly a disease of childhood. The condition may exist undetected for months or years, especially in institutions.

3. Marginal degeneration of cornea. A vascularized furrow, usually bilateral, running along the limbus and separated from it by a narrow clear zone. It may be superimposed on arcus senilis. A frequent sequela of this condition is ectasia or perforation. (Note ectasia as dark area on upper part of furrow.) Bacterial complication is particularly dangerous.

4. Rodent ulcer (Mooren's ulcer). A chronic, superficial corneal ulcer, of unknown etiology, occurring in the elderly. Laboratory diagnostic tests are negative. Simultaneously with the ulcer's advance, the peripheral portion of the lesion heals, with heavy vascularization.

5. Lye burn. A catastrophic occurrence in which liquefying necrosis (unlike coagulative necrosis from acid) develops rapidly, often within a few minutes.

6. This case showed abundant white discharge, with complete destruction of the conjunctiva and cornea. Even in apparently mild burns, destruction may later develop; cautious prognosis is advised. Laboratory diagnosis is mandatory to rule out bacterial infection.

7. Leukoma of the cornea, sequela of bacterial keratitis. Dark spot shows cystoid degeneration (usually resulting in fistula).

8. Multiple papilloma of the conjunctiva spreads over the fornix and slightly over the cornea. Superficial and benign, but it can show evidence of malignancy. It can be found in wearers of contact lenses.

Plate 41

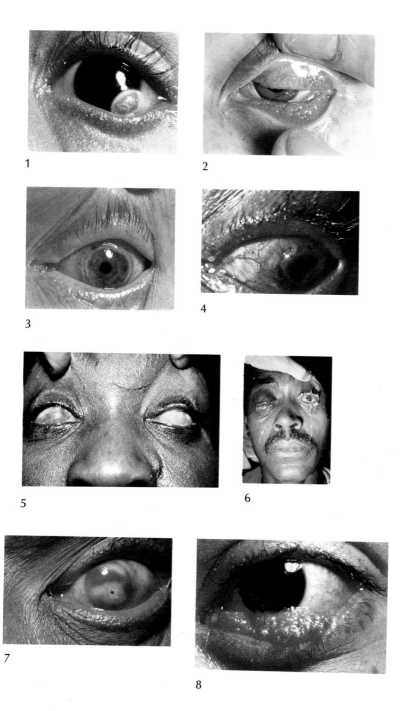

1

2

3

4

5

6

7

8

Plate 42

1, 2. Bowen's disease (two cases). Intraepithelial tumor—carcinoma in situ. Considerably vascularized, typically located at limbus and spread over cornea. Growth rapid and can metastasize. Often follows dyskeratosis. Can also be preceded by inflammation, trauma, or burn.

3. Lymphoma of conjunctiva often associated with generalized lymphomatous hyperplasia, particularly with acute or chronic leukemia.

4. Corneal tumorlike leproma extending to anterior eye and orbit. Ulceration rare. Hansen's bacilli can be found in corneal scraping.

5. Lid syphilides in male 24 years old (Parinuad's syndrome). Eruptions occurring on lid and elsewhere (lower). Lid margin destruction leaves a typical serpiginous deformity (upper).

6. Epithelioma of conjunctiva, usually epibulbar, superficially spreading over cornea and sclera. Highly vascuiarized and slow-growing tumor. Metastases may occur.

Plate   42

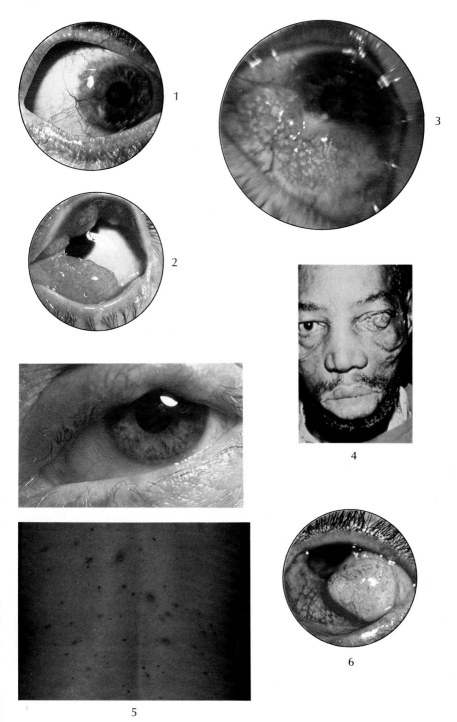

Plate 43

1. Good epithelium. Chromatin (nuclear) evenly distributed, nuclear and cytoplasmic border clear.

2. Columnar epithelium with abnormal tail of cytoplasm.

3. Goblet cells with pinkish clumps of mucoid material. Nucleus pushed toward cell membrane. (Courtesy Dr. R. A. Hyndiuk, University of Milwaukee.)

4. Epithelial tumor cells, characterized by extreme hyperchromasia. Variation in chromatin arrangement is most important criterion for malignancy—irregular, uneven distribution. Cytoplasm markedly varies in size (may be absent), distribution, and staining. Cells of carcinoma (Giemsa stain).

5. Squamous carcinoma cells (Papanicolaou stain). (Courtesy of Dr. M. Spinack, Montefiore Hospital Medical Center.)

6. Mascara deposit, concretionlike. Surrounding cells markedly degenerated.

7. Keratinization. Different stages depending entirely on nucleus: **A.** Prekeratinization, (precornification). Nucleus vesicular, cytoplasm basophilic. **B.** Keratinization, (cornification). Nucleus pyknotic with beginning caryorrhexis and acidophilic cytoplasm. **C.** Stage of keratin granules (not always present) resembling cells of stratum granulosum of epidermis. Study of keratinization is useful for differential diagnosis of allergy and infection.

Plate 43

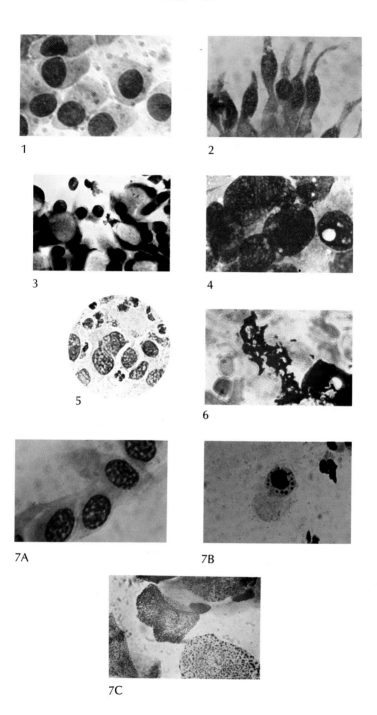

1

2

3

4

5

6

7A

7B

7C

Plate 44

1. Lymphocytic reaction: **A.** Lymphocytes, medium and large. Lympho-blast found in acute lymphatic reaction or chlamydial disease. **B.** Mature lymphocytes usually predominant in chronic inflammation or cell-mediated allergy. **C.** Pyknotic lymphocytes usually indicate toxic reaction. **D.** Plasma cells often increase in chlamydial diseases and cell-mediated allergy.

2. Mast cell and eosinophil found in allergy.

3. Monocytic cells: reticuloendothelial cells having a phagocytic function may be predominant in viral infection, particularly adenoviral. **A.** Large cells usually with bending nucleus (showing some pyknosis) and vacuolized large cytoplasm indicating ingestion. **B.** Monocytes with phagocytized neutrophil. **C.** Giant macrophage—Leber cell with phagocytized nuclear and cytoplasmic debris. More often found in chlamydial diseases.

Plate 44

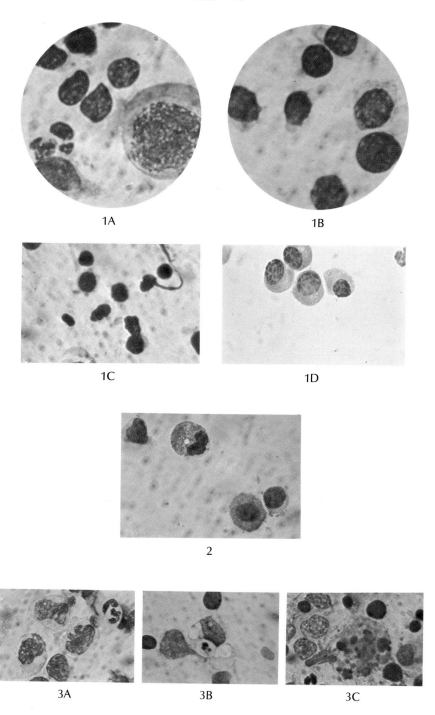

1A

1B

1C

1D

2

3A

3B

3C

Plate 45

1. A moistened swab is passed along the cul-de-sac after eversion of the lid.

2. After having streaked across plate with conjunctival swab, culture from lid margin with moistened applicator.

3. Streaking method for conjunctival and lid cultures (schematic).

4. Growth on blood agar after culturing conjunctiva and lid borders.

5. A support is placed behind the canaliculus, and pressure is applied anteriorly to obtain a sample from the canaliculus.

Plate   45

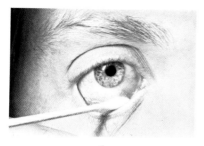

1

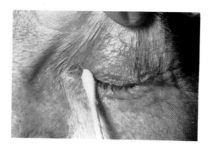

2

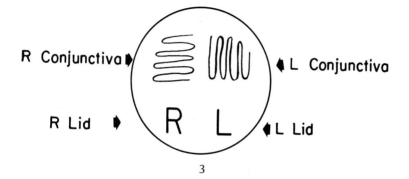

R Conjunctiva ▶   ◀ L Conjunctiva

R Lid ▶   ◀ L Lid

3

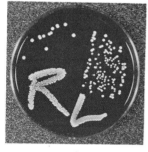

4

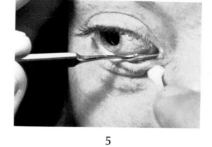

5

Plate 46

1. Firm pressure on the fundus of the lacrimal sac with an applicator will express material from the sac that can be secured from the punctum.

2. Biopsy specimen from suspected keratomycosis showing *Candida* pseudohyphae in stroma.

3. Chocolate agar plates in candle jar used to raise carbon dioxide concentration.

4. Scraping of corneal ulcer at leading edge and base, using *modified* Kimura spatula.

5. Modified Kimura spatula is narrower than standard Kimura spatula and is better able to debride and hold corneal specimens, especially when dealing with small ulcers.

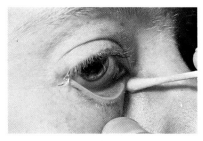

Plate 46

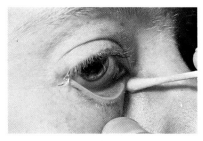

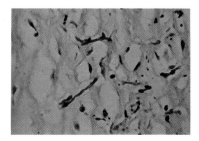

1

2

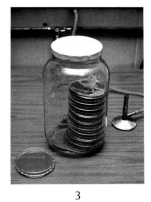

3

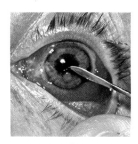

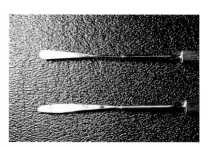

4

5

Plate 47

1. Corneal specimens are C-streaked. Growth on C is considered to be from the corneal ulcer, while growth off C streak is probably a contaminant.

2. Schematic guide to corneal ulcer work-up.

3. Scraping of conjunctiva with unmodified Kimura spatula so that conjunctiva is mildly blanched.

4. Material from conjunctival scraping should be spread firmly and evenly on a glass slide.

5. After scraping, slide should be immediately immersed into absolute methanol in a coplin jar.

Plate 47

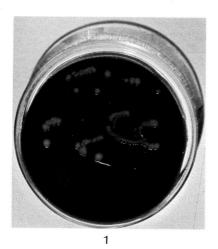

1

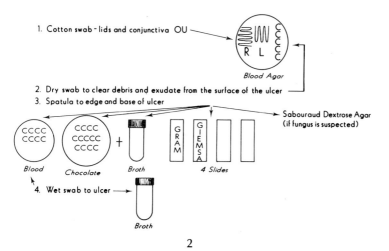

1. Cotton swab - lids and conjunctiva OU

Blood Agar

2. Dry swab to clear debris and exudate from the surface of the ulcer

3. Spatula to edge and base of ulcer

→ Sabouraud Dextrose Agar
(if fungus is suspected)

Blood   *Chocolate*   *Broth*   GRAM GIEMSA   *4 Slides*

4. Wet swab to ulcer   *Broth*

2

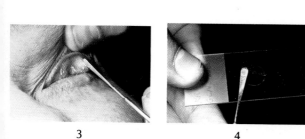

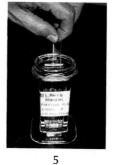

3   4   5

1

Bacterial External Infections of the Eye

Almost any pathogenic bacteria can cause ocular infection. Certain bacteria, such as *Moraxella lacunata*, *Corynebacterium xerosis*, and the Koch-Weeks bacillus (Weeks, 1886) *(Haemophilus aegyptius)*, (Cason; Berens, Nilson and Darrel) are usually ophthalmic.

The general principle that infection is determined chiefly by the virulence of the microorganisms and by host resistance applies to the eye. However, ocular infections have certain characteristics resulting from the unique anatomic structure, physiology, and biochemistry of the eye. Bacteria themselves, particularly opportunistic bacteria, may undergo some changes in the specific environment of the involved tissue.

Certain bacteria have a special affinity for specific ocular structures. For instance, infection by the gonococcus results in conjunctivitis, but the lacrimal apparatus is not involved, the Koch-Weeks bacillus *(H. aegyptius)* causes conjunctivitis but not primary keratitis, and *C. xerosis* can grow only on dead epithelium.

External bacterial infections of the eye are usually localized but may frequently spread to adjacent tissue, from the conjunctiva to the cornea or into the inner eye or to the orbit or even to the brain. This is particularly true of streptococcal infections. Some external ocular infections can even be the focus from which metastatic involvement of the body occurs (eg, infection with the meningococcus or the gonococcus).

Conjunctivitis. Numerous factors protect the conjunctiva from bacterial infection. Among these are (1) a flushing mechanism provided by tears, (2) the bactericidal action of lysozyme, which is found in tears, (3) phagocytosis, in which the epithelial cells also take part, and

97

(4) the mechanical barrier of an intact mucous membrane. Other factors, such as immunity, play an important role. The conjunctiva is an anatomic and physiologic defense barrier.

The conjunctiva, since it is exposed, is the part of the eye most frequently infected. It is sterile at birth but shortly thereafter becomes invaded with various saprophytic bacteria. *C. xerosis* and *Staphylococcus epidermidis* are regarded as its almost constant inhabitants. Other strains of *Staphylococcus*, *M. lacunata*, the pneumococcus, the Koch-Weeks bacillus, and even streptococci, meningococci, and other organisms may also be found in the so-called normal flora of the conjunctiva, but they may be considered potentially pathogenic. All of these, with the exception of *C. xerosis*, may become pathogenic at one time or another. The conjunctiva may harbor many bacteria and thus be a source of infection for other parts of the body or for other individuals. Meningococci are particularly dangerous, as they can lead to meningitis of the host or even to epidemics of meningitis.

The majority of conjunctival infections are bacterial or viral; fungal infections are rarer. The prevalence of specific types of bacteria varies in different processes. Pneumococci and *H. aegyptius* predominantly are found in acute conjunctivitis, and staphylococci are found in chronic conjunctivitis. The anatomic structure of the external eye plays the main role in the determination of the pathology. Eruptions, ulcers, and abscesses are not typical for the conjunctiva, the most common manifestation being conjunctivitis, acute and chronic.

The inflammatory conjunctival response to infection is principally of two types: (1) exudative (discharge) and (2) productive (follicles or papillary hypertrophy).

EXUDATIVE CONJUNCTIVITIS.   The exudate, whether purulent, fibrinous, or hemorrhagic, is usually mixed with mucus and is not exclusively characteristic of a particular bacterial species. The purulent exudate is typically caused by pyogenic bacteria, such as staphylococci and neisseria, and some viruses, eg, vaccinia, smallpox, and others, and is usually a bilateral process. If purulent conjunctivitis is chronic and unilateral, the lacrimal passages can be affected, and it is then known as "lacrimal conjunctivitis." The fibrinous exudate, clinically manifested as pseudomembranous or membranous conjunctivitis, is chiefly caused by *Corynebacterium diphtheriae*, hemolytic streptococci, adenovirus, or hypersensitivity. Chronic membranous conjunctivitis with no known etiology has presented a problem for many years. However, membranes can be found in any severe acute conjunctivitis. Hemorrhagic exudation or petechiae possibly indicate hypersensitive reaction to infection. Acute conjunctivitis with exudation is called "catarrhalis" and is usually a self-limited process of a duration of about two weeks. Staphylococcal conjunctivitis has a tendency to become chronic.

Since bacterial conjunctivitis is typically an exudative process, the discharge is its most characteristic feature and is the source of transmission of infection.

Secondary corneal involvement may occur in any conjunctivitis. The keratitis is typically marginal and is believed to be the result of bacterial allergy or toxin and not caused by the bacteria themselves. This keratitis is usually not serious and resolves with healing of the conjunctiva. Marginal keratitis is mainly associated with staphylococcal infection.

The epithelial type of keratitis is almost always present in any acute bacterial conjunctivitis. The corneal epithelium is a continuation of the conjunctival epithelium. Therefore its involvement may be considered a part of the conjunctivitis. The epithelial type of keratitis must be differentiated from several superficial punctate keratitides of obscure etiology.

The type of exudate, corneal·complication, and severity of infection are influenced to a great extent by hygiene, nutrition, and other factors. In certain geographic areas, bacterial conjunctivitis is found to be chiefly purulent with abundant discharge, and it is often associated with secondary keratitis, which may be severe.

PRODUCTIVE CONJUNCTIVITIS.   The conjunctiva reacts to any kind of irritation by developing lymphatic hyperplasia and by the formation of follicles. Follicles are not seen in the bulbar conjunctiva, but they are sometimes seen at the limbus. This occurs in cases of poor hygiene, malnutrition, metabolic disturbances, and errors of refraction, particularly in hyperopia. It is a common reaction and by no means distinctive.

In the newborn, true lymphatic tissue develops at the age of three to four months after birth and reaches a maximum in 6 years. Therefore neonatal conjunctivitis is not follicular but usually purulent, regardless of the causative agent. However, pseudomembranes or true membranes can be found in acute conjunctivitis, whatever the etiology.

Children, especially those with lymphadenopathy, are particularly prone to the development of folliculosis. This process is not inflammatory and is called by some "adenoids of the conjunctiva." It can be so massive as to be mistaken for lymphoma (Plate 42, Fig. 3).

Follicular conjunctivitis can be either acute or chronic. The acute form is almost pathognomonic of such viruses as adenovirus, herpesvirus, influenza virus A, Newcastle disease virus, varicella-zoster virus, and cat-scratch fever virus but is unusual in the common cold, smallpox, or vaccinia. Coxsackie B1 viral conjunctivitis has developed in a laboratory worker.

Hyperacute follicular conjunctivitis is often found in patients overtreated with antibiotics. Multiple corneal erosion, pannus, and sometimes heavy scarring (shrinkage) may result. The mechanism is not clear.

Chronic follicular conjunctivitis is commonly found in trachoma, with some allergies, after the continued use of mascara, or in chronic follicular conjunctivitis of Axenfeld of unknown etiology.

Productive conjunctivitis can also be papillary. The structure of the papilla is different from that of the follicle. It has vessels in the center, surrounded by connective tissue and a hyperplastic epithelium. In follicles the vessels are peripheral, and there is no hyperplasia of the epithelium. Follicles are the aggregation of lymphocytes, large and young in the center, and small and mature in the periphery. Follicles are spheroid in form and yellowish in color, whereas papillae are red and flat. The location is different also, follicles usually starting at the fornix and papillae at the tarsal conjunctiva (Plate 22, Fig. 2).

Papillary hypertrophy is usually found in chronic conjunctivitis of the aged and is the result of prolonged hyperemia and neovascularization. It is also found in the resultant stage of purulent conjunctivitis and in the later stage of trachoma, tuberculosis, vernal conjunctivitis, contact allergy, syphilis, and leprosy.

The increasing number of patients with dry eyes is becoming a serious problem, not only among aged patients but also as a result of the wide use of steroids, dehydrating drugs, contact lenses, and mascara. Follicular or papillary reaction may occur.

Blepharitis.   The lid margin is the meeting place of three layers: the cutaneous, the tarsal, and the conjunctival. It is a densely packed area with modified sebaceous, meibomian, and Zeis glands, the sweat glands of Moll, and cilia. Therefore, lid margins are the most common site of pathology of the eye. Important in the development of blepharitis is the fact that the lid margin acts as an extremity, and such circulatory disturbances as stasis often occur. Blond or anemic persons with sensitive skin or individuals with highly vascularized skin can easily develop red-rimmed eyes. While this in itself is not a diseased condition, it may predispose to blepharitis. There is sensitivity to minor irritants, the chief complaint being itching, and various irritants, both endogenous and exogenous, may cause hyperemia. If the irritation persists, stasis occurs, metabolic products collect, and autosensitization may result. In this favorable situation, bacteria grow readily.

Another factor of importance in the development of blepharitis is that the lashes act as receptacles for dust and bacteria, providing a favorable environment for infection. Of all the organisms, staphylococci are the prime offenders.

Blepharitis is characterized by chronicity and may even last a lifetime. It is subject to troublesome recurrences. The mechanism of chronic and recurrent inflammation is unknown, but there is increased belief that the antigen–antibody complex plays an important role. The lid margins become rounded and thickened (tylosis ciliaris). The lashes fall out because of hair follicle destruction (madarosis), or the lid margins may become deformed, especially in older persons, resulting in trichiasis or ectropion. There may be tear film dysfunction. As a result the cornea is more exposed to injury, dryness, and superficial punctate keratis (SPK), or marginal keratitis often develops.

Staphylococcal blepharitis is usually associated with an acute or chronic meibomitis. The organisms are harbored in the glands, which act as reservoirs for prolonged infection or sensitization.

Since the condition occurs in poor hygienic surroundings and in persons whose resistance is low, the main objectives of treatment must be improvement of general health and cleanliness of the eye. Removal of scales and crusts before further treatment is mandatory. The patient should wash his face at least twice a day with hot water and soap.

Seborrheic blepharitis is even more troublesome and more frequent than is staphylococcal blepharitis. Hypersecretion of the sebaceous glands in seborrhea is usually generalized. In older persons, it may be a local process, either hypersecretion or atonic retention of the meibomian glands. The normal cholesterol fats change to cholesterol esters, which support growth, particularly of *Pityrosporum ovale* and staphylococci. These organisms aggravate the seborrheic blepharitis, which then may become ulcerative. If this does not occur, seborrheic blepharitis is a mild process characterized by greasy scales. The foamy secretion along the lid margin is a sign of hypersecretion of the meibomian glands.

The expression of the secretion, simultaneously with massage, has primary importance in treatment. The patient, properly instructed, can do it himself.

Keratitis.   The cornea is a unique anatomic structure. It consists of a hard, homogeneous, avascular tissue which is incapable of regeneration, except for epithelial cells and Descemet's membrane. The predominant feature of corneal infection is a necrosis, often with resulting ulcer formation. Damage, unless extremely mild, leaves a permanent mark on the cornea.

There are two main types of keratitis in which bacteria have to be considered: marginal and central hypopyon. Marginal keratitis (Thygeson, 1948), while common in bacterial conjunctivitis and blepharitis, is rarely caused by the bacteria themselves but is rather a secondary toxic or hypersentivity response. This form of keratitis is not severe and usually heals at the same time as the conjunctivitis.

Central infectious keratitis generally follows corneal trauma and is due to direct invasion by infectious agents. The process is severe and destructive and can end with endophthalmitis and panophthalmitis. It can even be a focus for metastatic sepsis, particularly with streptococci and gonococci. The severity of the process depends upon three major factors: (1) the virulence of the invasive organism, (2) the position of the infection, and (3) the debility of the patient.

The central part of the cornea is most exposed, most sensitive, thinnest, and, above all, most poorly nourished and poorly supplied by antibodies. Central infectious keratitis is usually purulent, and an infiltration of a yellowish color is characteristic. It is accompanied by a sterile hypopyon, which indicates that toxin penetrates into the anterior chamber, causing iritis. There is a purulent conjunctivitis secondary to the keratitis.

In the preantibiotic era, the common organism in central hypopyon keratitis was the pneumococcus. Now gram-negative bacilli, particularly of the enteric group, are the main agents of this disease. New infectious strains have arisen that were formerly considered nonpathogenic. These are known as "opportunistic organisms" and are highly resistant to antibiotics. We are now beginning to recognize anaerobes as a major source of serious infection, particularly in drug addicts.

At Bellevue Hospital, a high incidence of moraxella keratitis, particularly in alcoholics, has decreased markedly, probably due to improvement in the social conditions of alcoholics.

In addition to the bacterial infections are the fungal corneal ulcers, which will be considered in Chapter 4.

The prognosis for central purulent keratitis is always guarded, particularly in that caused by gram-negative bacilli and by fungi, most of which are resistant to antibiotics.

Another type of severe purulent infectious keratitis is the ring abscess, which is usually metastatic in origin and is found in dysentery, urinary tract infections, diabetes, and other infections.

Purulent keratitis can be aseptic.

There are many other types of keratitis associated with infections, the vascular type, pannus—classical in trachoma—some viral infections such as molluscum contagiosum, and in the allergic phlyctenular process.

Deep interstitial keratitis, diffuse or in sector, vascular or avascular, is not typically ulcerative. It is found in viral and bacterial infections, tuberculosis, and syphilis.

Dacryocystitis.   The basis for this infection is a blockage of the lacrimal duct system, and the process is usually unilateral. The flushing mechanism is disturbed, and tear fluid collects in the lacrimal sac. The tears, which have served to clear the eye, wash the bacteria into the sac, where they may readily multiply. Among the microorganisms, often mixed, that may be found are staphylococci, streptococci, *Branhamella (Neisseria) catarrhalis*, *H. aegyptius*, *Pseudomonas aeruginosa*, and others. The pneumococcus is the most common inhabitant. Fungal infections, such as aspergillosis, *Candida albicans*, blastomycosis, and sporotrichosis (resembling tuberculosis), have increased in this antibiotic era.

Two main types of dacryocystitis exist: chronic and acute. Chronic dacryocystitis is "silent," symptomless. Chronic unilateral purulent conjunctivitis can be the key to its diagnosis, and expression of the exudate is important in diagnosis. Chronic dacryocystitis is easy to overlook, and the result can be disastrous, with postoperative infection or hypopyon keratitis.

Acute dacryocystitis may develop from chronic dacryocystitis if the inner wall of the sac is injured. It is usually very severe, involving the perilacrimal tissue (cellulitis). The expression of its exudate is inhibited by blockage of the canaliculi, and the etiologic diagnosis is difficult. If the infection does not resolve under medical management or if hypopyon keratitis develops, surgical procedures are necessary.

Neonatal dacryocystitis is due to blockage of the lacrimal ducts by the unobliterated membrane or to the accumulation of exfoliated epithelium mixed with exudate. The exudate is purulent but usually sterile. It is recommended by most authorities that probing should not be done before a child is one year old (Plate 3, Fig. 6).

2

Bacteria

MORPHOLOGIC CHARACTERISTICS OF BACTERIA

EXTERNAL STRUCTURE

Cell Wall. This is the rigid outer layer of the bacterium. Chemically, it consists of proteins, carbohydrates, and lipids.

Cytoplasmic Membrane. This is the concentrated peripheral part of the cytoplasm, adjacent to the inner surface of the cell wall.

Being semipermeable membranes, the cell wall and the cytoplasmic membrane both serve as osmotic barriers between the external and internal environments of the bacterial cell. These structures have many other characteristics, such as antigenic properties and electric charge (tendency of bacteria to migrate in an electric field).

Capsule. This superficial slime layer surrounds the bacterial cell wall (it appears as a clear zone, especially in stained preparation). It is suggested that, depending upon environment, practically all bacteria can develop capsules. The degree of encapsulation differs. Some bacteria have a well-developed capsule, while others have an almost invisible one. However, in certain bacteria, capsules are constantly present, probably a heredity characteristic. Some bacteria develop a capsule only in tissue (eg, *Clostridium perfringens*), while some develop capsules in both tissue and culture (the pneumococcus and *Klebsiella pneumoniae*).

Chemically, the capsular material is not a permanent structure. In many species, the capsule consists of polysaccharides, which stimulate the formation of antibodies in tissues. In certain groups of pneumococci, *K. pneumoniae,* and *Haemophilus influenzae,* the capsular carbohydrates also determine the specificity of the serologic groups. Medical

104

bacteriologists correlate the presence of a capsule with virulence (the capsule serves as a means of protection for the pathogens, mainly against phagocytosis).

Flagella.   These are the organs of motion. Some bacteria are able to move throughout their life, and others are motile only during certain periods of cell development. Flagella are cytoplasmic processes extending through the pores in the cell wall and chemically composed of proteins. They are very thin, are usually longer than the cell body, and are arranged in various patterns on the bacterial cell, one or more in number.

A number of bacteria (most bacilli, spirilla, and some coccal forms, particularly saprophytic) have flagella. Not all motile bacteria move by means of flagella. Spirochetes seem to swim like snakes. There is no relationship between flagellar motility and tissue invasion or pathogenicity in general.

The active motion also can be due to impulses originating within the bacteria themselves.

INTERNAL STRUCTURE

Nucleus.   Opinions regarding the presence of a nucleus in bacteria have ranged from complete denial that a bacterial nucleus exists to the assumption that the entire bacterial cell is a nucleus. The process of transmission of hereditary factors in bacteria confirms the existence of nuclear material. Demonstration of a bacterial nucleus is difficult because most bacteria contain large amounts of ribonucleic acid (RNA), which masks the real nucleic material-deoxyribonucleic acid (DNA), because RNA has the same high sensitivity to basic dyes as does DNA. After the removal of RNA by the enzyme ribonuclease, the Feulgen reaction, which is specific for DNA, is often positive in bacterial structures. These structures do not show a nucleus typical of that of higher organisms. They do not have typical chromosomes, and they multiply not by mitosis but by simple division of the nucleus into two daughter fragments. However, on the basis of recent data, the presence of chromosomes is assumed.

Cytoplasmic Elements.   Bacterial cytoplasm is a structureless colloidal mixture of enzymes and metabolites with a variety of granules.

VOLUTIN GRANULES.   These are also known as metachromatic granules, Babes-Ernst granules, and ribonucleic acid granules. Common in most bacteria, they occur in the form of refractile granules having the same high affinity to basic dyes as does chromatin material. Because volutin granules are not a permanent structure and may disappear completely after starvation of bacteria, they are regarded as food storage for bacteria. The presence of volutin granules is significant for diagnosis and for differentiation of bacterial species, particularly *Corynebacterium* species.

CARBOHYDRATES.   Reserve polysaccharide-glycogen and starch granules are found in many bacterial species. They may be regarded as food storage. The granules are identified by staining with iodine.

FATS AND LIPIDS.   Fat globules are a common finding in bacteria, being particularly abundant in acid-fast bacilli. The very refractile and intensely stained fat globules resemble chromatin material or endospores.

Spores.   Sporulation of bacteria generally occurs in an unfavorable environment (eg, a dry one). As soon as spores again find good conditions they germinate into fresh vegetative cells. Spores are seen in unstained films as highly refractive spherical bodies surrounded by light zones. They may be seen in stained films only when spore membranes are permeable. Most yeasts, molds, and many bacilli produce spores, while most cocci do not. Usually only a single spore develops, occasionally two. In some bacteria *(Clostridium)* the spores cause a bulge. Filamentous bacteria (eg, *Nocardia*) may produce spores termed "conidia," which very closely resemble the spores of molds.

Chemically, spores are rich in lipids and apparently contain a large amount of chromatinlike nuclear material.

Size.   Next to viruses and rickettsia, bacteria are the smallest living organisms, and this is their most characteristic property. There is great variation in size (range: 0.1 to 50 μ), but the majority of bacteria studied in the laboratory are between 0.5 and 2 μ. Size is influenced by heredity and environmental factors.

Size has a great effect on the behavior of bacteria. Volume and surface area are important factors in the process of diffusion and elimination of waste products. The smaller the bacteria, the less complex is their structure, and they are apt to be deficient in enzymes and, hence, more dependent upon the host cells. The antigenic properties of smaller bacteria have a more specific action.

The larger species of a genus have a lower temperature growth range than do the small ones. A bacterial population that has passed beyond the stage of its maximum growth rate consists of smaller bacteria than are found in a young culture. Only corynebacteria are smaller in young culture.

Size is the main determining factor in the segmentation of bacteria. As the bulk of a bacterium increases, the surface becomes proportionately smaller, and the necessity arises for segmentation or subdivision of the organism.

Shape.   Three main morphologic groups are recognized: coccal or spheroidal (including lancet-shaped, flattened, and kidney-shaped), bacillary, ·filamentous, cylindrical, and spiral. The variety of shapes may be very marked. Bacillary, coccal, and filamentous forms may all be present in the same species, which is then called "pleomorphic." Age, environment, species, and even the technique of preparing the specimen are important determinants of shape.

Grouping or Arrangement. When a bacterial cell divides, the two daughter cells may remain attached to one another by their cell membrane, or they may separate immediately. Depending on the plane and the number of divisions and the tendency to remain together, various arrangements occur. It is a general rule that the division of bacteria takes place at a right angle to the longest axis of the cell—it is transverse, not longitudinal. In cocci, the division may occur in any plane, since a sphere has no longest axis. As a result, cocci show a greater variety of grouping than do bacilli. Among the cocci the diplo or strepto arrangement is the result of parallel division, tetra is the result of division in two planes, sarcine in three planes, and cluster results from irregular division. Among the bacilli, which are always divided perpendicularly to their long axis, the arrangement occurs typically in diplobacillary and streptobacillary forms. The chain arrangement in bacilli has no inference of pathogenicity, as it does in cocci formation. In some bacteria *(Corynebacterium)* a postfission movement occurs which can bring the cells into parallel or palisade arrangement or at an angle (in L, V, or T shapes or as Chinese letters).

Since the grouping of bacteria may be much influenced by physical and mechanical factors in the environment, arrangement itself is not sufficiently significant for diagnosis. However, in combination with typical shape and staining, arrangement may be of determinative value.

Reproduction. This can occur during the active vegetative or resting stage. The usual method of multiplication is by simple binary fission, which occurs as a transverse, never longitudinal, segmentation of bacteria. In addition to fission other methods of multiplication include sporulation, budding, and sexual reproduction. Spores are reproductive bodies. The sexual type of reproduction (the fusion of two cells) is relatively primitive, due to the primitive structure of the nucleus.

HOST–PARASITE RELATIONSHIP

A great variety of factors characterizes the ability of a microorganism to establish disease in a given host. It is impossible to mention all of them, even briefly.

The most important principle is that the infectious agent must be able to penetrate the protective cellular and humoral barriers of the host and to find a favorable environment for multiplication. To destroy the protective barrier, the infectious agent must be virulent. Virulence is determined by a great number of complex factors. Most important among these are invasiveness and toxigenicity.

Invasiveness. Many diseases develop not because of toxin but primarily because of invasiveness—the ability of microorganisms to enter the body. They multiply locally in tissue and spread easily via the lymphatics to the bloodstream, causing bacteremia (eg, anthrax and plague bacilli invade tissue rapidly and multiply extensively in most tissues).

ENZYMES.   These play a leading role in the process of invasiveness, although knowledge of their action is incomplete. A brief description of some enzymes will ·be given.

Collagenase is a proteolytic enzyme that disintegrates collagen, helping the spread of infection in tissue. It is produced by C. *perfringens*, pseudomonas, and others.

Hyaluronidase is a spreading factor that hydrolyzes hyaluronic acid, a cementing substance of tissue. It also hydrolyzes a capsular component of certain bacteria.

Streptokinase is a proteolytic enzyme produced mainly by certain hemolytic streptococci. It dissolves human fibrin clots, in indirect action. It is believed that streptokinase activates plasminogen, which is a precursor of plasmin, a proteolytic ferment in plasma.

Streptodornase is a streptococcal deoxyribonuclease enzyme that lowers the viscosity of DNA. The viscosity of purulent exudate depends largely upon the deoxyribonuclease proteins.

Coagulase coagulates plasma to form a wall around staphylococcal lesions. It also protects staphylococci from phagocytosis by a deposit of fibrin on the surface of the bacteria.

A number of toxic and nontoxic substances are elaborated by pathogenic bacteria during their growth. These are hemolysin, fibrinolysin, leukocidin, erythrogenic toxin, and others.

Toxigenicity.   Toxins are subdivided into exotoxins and endotoxins.

Exotoxins are liberated into surrounding tissues by many gram-positive (rarely gram-negative) bacteria. They have a specific effect on certain cells of the host (eg, tetanus toxin affects motor nerve cells). Exotoxins stimulate the production of antibodies in amounts proportional to the toxin and are specifically neutralized by them. They can also be converted into toxoids (antigenic but nonpoisonous) by heat, formalin, and prolonged storage.

Endotoxins are intimately associated with most gram-negative bacteria. They can be liberated into the surrounding medium only by autolysis of the bacteria (not by simple filtration). They are weakly toxic, and high doses are needed to produce diseases in experimental animals. They are unstable and do not produce fever, and they do not stimulate the formation of antitoxins. Chemically, endotoxins are lipid-polysaccharide, identical to the O antigen, type-specific of enteric bacilli, found in the bodies of bacteria, and equally efficient in the production of antibodies as a whole bacterium.

Endotoxins of most gram-negative bacilli are similar, as are their pharmacologic and pathologic effects. Therefore, the existence of a common toxic component is assumed.

The majority of gram-negative bacilli are strongly resistant to most antibiotics.

In the ability of a parasite to produce infection, a variety of other factors play important roles. The route of introduction of the infectious agent modifies the virulence (very toxic tetanus is harmless when swallowed; many bacteria nonpathogenic in intact tissue become very virulent in injured tissue). The site of the primary lesion and the direction of initial spread of infection, particularly by the direction of lymphatic flow, are largely determined by the portal of entry. However, the biochemical environment of the host tissue (resistance and immunity) (Leopold et al) ultimately determines the production of infection.

Resistance and Immunity.   Resistance is determined by humoral and cellular defense barriers of the host, in which two groups of factors must be considered: nonspecific and specific.

NONSPECIFIC FACTORS.   Anatomic defense barriers are intact skin and mucous membranes. Some bacteria may penetrate these structures, and others may be introduced by arthropods. Intact epithelium is a defense against the entry of bacteria, and epithelial trauma is very important in the development of infection, particularly in tissue with a low grade of resistance. Whereas superficial trauma is insignificant for the conjunctiva, it is serious in the cornea. Erosion of the conjunctiva is an almost unknown diagnosis but a very significant one for the cornea.

Physiologic barriers are provided by the glands. There are numerous kinds of glands in both skin and mucous membranes. Sweat and fatty substances of acid pH have antimicrobial properties, and glands may play a negative role as a portal of entry for infection. Abscess formation of the skin is very common, though not typical for the conjunctiva.

Some bacteria have a preferred selection of tissue, eg, the gonococcus grows best in the genitourinary tract and the conjunctiva; *Corynebacterium diphtheriae* grows on the upper respiratory tract.

Skin resistance varies with age. The skin of children and of the elderly is more susceptible than that of adolescents. In the first month of an infant's life coliform bacterial infection often develops. It is believed that IgM and IgA, which have bactericidal effects on these bacteria, have failed to cross the placenta and have not yet developed in the infant.

PHAGOCYTOSIS.   Many microorganisms elaborate chemotactic factors attracting phagocytes. The cellular theory of phagocytosis was proposed by Metchnikoff in 1845. Phagocytosis is more active in the presence of opsonin. Phagocytes are either fixed (reticuloendothelial cells) or free (leukocytes).

Phagocytic macrophages (polymorphonuclear leukocytes) engulf the bacteria and, by their proteolytic ability, clean the debris.

Other phagocytes are (1) tissue cells, such as sessile, and (2) wandering monocytes in the tissue space or in the blood circulation. Aschoff gave both of these the name reticuloendothelial (RE) system, the function of which is to fight agents such as viruses, allergens, and small bacteria. The response is characterized by mononuclear cells. However, for some bacteria, phagocytosis is protective rather than destructive. The tubercle and leprosy bacilli can live and even multiply inside phagocytic cells. Two nonphagocytic cells, lymphocytes and plasma cells, have recently been added to the RE system.

Vascularization supplies different kinds of fluid, leukocytes, and antibodies in defense of the host. Therefore in the avascular cornea, lens, and vitreous, the defense mechanism is poor.

Corticosteroids diminish the phagocytic defense against bacterial and fungal infection.

SPECIFIC FACTORS.   The antigen-antibody reaction is the best known principal mechanism of immunity. However, cellular immunity is more important in preventing the development of a fatal infection.

Antigens are macromolecules with high molecular weight. They elicit antibody formation and have these characteristics: (1) protein antigens are complete antigens but must be foreign (nonself), (2) lipids and polysaccharides are usually incomplete antigens, (3) haptens are of low molecular weight (simple chemicals or drugs) and are able to elicit antibody formation only after combining with body proteins or other antibodies.

Antibodies (1) react specifically with the antigen that stimulates their production, (2) are produced in lymphatic tissue in plasma cells (Allansmith et al; Savage et al), (3) are specialized serum immunoglobulins of five types: IgG, IgA, IgM, IgD, and IgE (Allansmith et al). The newborn is protected by IgG maternal antibodies for the first few months of life.

In the eye, only the lens has no immunoglobulins. It is possible that many eye diseases are antibody-dependent.

The humoral antigen–antibody reaction was known as a simple immunologic system. In recent years intensive experimental study in ocular immunology (Allansmith et al; Aronson et al; Kaufman, Silverstein et al; Silverstein) showed the important immunologic role of the cellular system, which also includes immune competence and immunologic memory. The cellular system is operative in the mediation of allergy because of the function of small lymphocytes.

Functionally, there are T lymphocytes and B lymphocytes. T lymphocytes are derived from the thymus gland. They live a long life, contributing to immunologic memory, and memory cells can transfer cellular immunity in the absence of humoral immunity. T lymphocytes do not produce antibodies but are responsible for the cell-mediated allergy-delayed type of immunity. B lymphocytes are produced by bone marrow, spleen, liver, and possibly the lymphatic tissue of the intestines. They are a smaller part of serum lymphocytes than are T cells, and their life is short. Their main function is the production of antibodies.

Since certain diseases are mediated and transferred by lymphocytes (Ezra), the principle of antilymphatic treatment is gaining acceptance. The immunologic role of eosinophils, unknown before, was recently studied, and there is evidence that eosinophils secrete inhibitors to inflammation. They play a part in local humoral and cellular defense mechanism by their inhibitors.

Immunity may be natural or acquired, active or passive.

HYPERSENSITIVITY

The distinction between the terms "hypersensitivity" and "allergy" is quantitative rather than qualitative. In many infections, the allergic state plays an important and dominant role, clinically and pathologically. Allergy can be roughly divided into immediate and delayed types. However, these are not always sharply distinguishable.

The delayed (cell-mediated) reaction is common in most diseases, including bacterial, and develops within no less than 12 to 48 hours and progresses for two to three days, or longer. There is no circulating antibody in serum, and it can be transferred only by cells (lymphoid) or their extract. The inflammatory reaction is characterized not by prominent edema but by mononuclear infiltration and tissue induration. Eosinophils are rarely found.

The tuberculin reaction is a classical type of delayed allergy. A tuberculinlike sensitivity may be induced by almost any type of protein. Delayed allergy occurs more frequently in certain chronic infections—bacterial, viral, or fungal. Spontaneous sensitization of this type occurs regularly in tuberculosis, typhoid, glanders, brucellosis,

pneumococcal pneumonia, chancroid, echinococcal infection, streptococcal infection, lymphogranuloma venereum, coccidioidomycosis, histoplasmosis, mumps, and vaccinia viral infection.

Bacterial infection may be complicated by either immediate or delayed sensitivity, which is termed "bacterial allergy."

The delayed type of allergy is recognized in many conditions other
than infections and is usually manifested as a dermatitis, such as contact dermatitis. The classical example of this is dermatitis due to contact
with poison ivy. Certain drugs and many chemicals used in manufac-
turing processes produce contact dermatitis. In many of these cases,
antigens are incomplete or haptens. Delayed hypersensitivity may play
a major part in the majority of eye allergies—conjunctivitis, keratitis,
blepharitis, uveitis, and others. This can occur after the use of certain
antibiotics, particularly neomycin and the sulfa drugs.

The immediate reaction, antibody-mediated, may develop within
two or three minutes and disappears within one hour (often several
hours). The reaction is usually acute and systemic and characterized by
prominent edema and erythema due to dilatation of capillaries and ar-
terioles. Cellular reaction is limited, and eosinophils may be present. It
is mediated by an antibody that can be circulated in serum and can be
transferred passively. Anaphylaxis and serum sickness are the classical
immediate reactions, and both are systemic. Allergy to pollen, some
allergies to antibiotics, and asthma are examples. It is usually an atopic
type of allergy with a family history.

The Arthus phenomenon is also an example of local immediate
reaction, which depends on high levels of precipitating antibody of the
IgG type. Examples in the human being are not well worked out.

The antigens present during fetal and neonatal life are recognized
as self and are tolerated by the host. The antigens not present in these
periods are nonself. Tolerance to self antigens may be lost, and an immunologic reaction to host antigens develops, bringing about autoimmune diseases. Autoimmune reactions may be involved in many general and eye diseases (Brown et al).

In allergic conditions predisposing factors—hunger, thirst, heat,
cold, fatigue, hygiene, and resistance of the host—must be considered.

GRAM–POSITIVE GROUP

PYOGENIC COCCI

The Staphylococci

Staphylococcus is a genus of the family Micrococcaceae. Staphylococci are actual or potential pathogens, being constant inhabitants of

the skin and most mucous membranes, including the conjunctiva. They produce a variety of infections, ranging from a mild carbuncle to fatal septicemia. Primarily a causative agent of pyogenic infections, staphylococci also have the ability to necrotize tissue and are usually characterized by abscess formation. Any structure of the body can be invaded by staphylococci. Staphylococci occupy first place among all organisms involved in ocular infections. Many strains have developed resistance to penicillin by producing penicillinase, an enzyme that destroys penicillin (Locatcher-Khorazo et al). Hospital staffs and patients carry these so-called hospital strains. They cause epidemics of infections that were unknown before the antibiotic era. The most endangered areas in hospitals are the nurseries for the newborn and the operating room.

Staphylococcal infections are usually sporadic, not epidemic, and their chronicity presents a difficult problem for treatment. Since the staphylococcus is a constant inhabitant of the skin and mucous membranes, the question arises regarding its etiologic significance in chronic recurrent diseases. The answer is based upon the number of organisms in smears and of colonies in cultures and the production of pigment, exotoxins, and enzymes, including the hemolysins.

Staphylococcal strains resistant to penicillin isolated from hospital patients and personnel have increased. As a result, some infections, such as staphylococcal enteritis, have become highly fatal.

Morphology. Staphylococci are typically gram-positive, extracellular, spherical, arranged in clusters, and do not possess a capsule (Plate 1, Fig. 5A). However, they vary in size, shape, and staining characteristics. In smear of the secretion, they can be intracellular, flattened on one side, and arranged singly, in pairs, or in short chains (Plate 1, Fig. 5B). There is also individual variation in resistance to decoloration by the gram method of staining, causing gram-negative cells to appear in some cultures. Because of these variations, diagnosis from direct smear is often impossible. Diagnosis is feasible only in cases where there are typical morphologic characteristics, such as spherical shape, definite gram-positive stain, and cluster arrangement. Culture is always necessary to confirm diagnosis and to test virulence and sensitivity.

Culture. Staphylococci grow readily on all ordinary bacteriologic media, and their colonies are easily identified on solid media. They are typically opaque, round, discrete (not mucoid), smooth, raised, glistening, and from 1 to 2 mm in diameter (Plate 1, Fig. 6). In smear from the culture, the morphology varies depending on whether the medium is solid or fluid, or the culture young or old.

The colonies show active pigment production. In the presence of oxygen, pigment production is enhanced, especially on agar containing carbohydrates. Also to be noted is that an incubation temperature of 22

C is more conducive to pigment production than is the usual incubation temperature of 37 C.

Pigment production varies in the three species now recognized: (1) *Staphylococcus aureus* produces mostly orange colonies, with some yellow colonies produced by antibiotic-resistant strains, (2) *Staphylococcus epidermidis* colonies are usually white or yellow, occasionally orange, and rarely purple, (3) *Staphylococcus saprophyticus* produces mostly white but occasionally yellow or orange colonies.

However, pigment production has less value than do results of the coagulase test in determining pathogenicity. It was once considered that *S. aureus* was the only pathogenic species of this genus, but it has now been shown that *S. epidermidis* can cause serious infection (Valenton and Okumoto). Tests for pathogenicity of staphylococci include fermentation of mannitol (Plate 2, Fig. 4), liquefaction of gelatin, and production of coagulase. The coagulase test is most conclusive for pathogenicity. However, bacterial endocarditis and even septicemia can be caused by coagulase-negative strains.

On blood agar, staphylococci may produce hemolysis, which is apparently not concerned directly with pathogenicity, as is the case with streptococcal hemolysis.

The virulence of pathogenic strains is generally, but not always, diminished by prolonged cultivation. Even after years of subculture in the laboratory the virulence may remain intact. Animal passage may enhance the virulence of the pathogenic strains, but it has not induced virulence in saprophytic strains. Many staphylococci found in man are not pathogenic for animals.

COAGULASE TEST. The technique for performing the coagulase test can be simplified as follows: citrated plasma is mixed on a microscope slide with a suspension of staphylococci. If the strain is pathogenic the suspension becomes coagulated (Plate 2, Fig. 3).

Staphylococci are hardy microorganisms in spite of the fact that they are not sporeformers. Staphylococci can be dried and still reproduce.

TOXINS AND ENZYMES. Most of the pathogenic staphylococci produce various toxins. They are (1) lethal toxins causing death of animals when injected intravenously, (2) leukocidin, destroying leukocytes (its role in pathogenicity is uncertain), (3) enterotoxin, causing acute gastroenteritis (food poisoning), and (4) others.

Coagulase, an enzyme produced by staphylococci, coagulates fibrin. This forms a wall around the individual staphylococci and around the lesions. Hence phagocytosis is prevented, and a limited abscess usually develops. There are many other extracellular substances, among them hyaluronidase (spreading factor), proteinase, and lipase.

Toxoid may be readily prepared from staphylococcal exotoxins. It stimulates antibody formation and is used in treatment. Toxoid may diminish the severity of infection, but there is no evidence that it can cure, and vaccine has an even more questionable value.

Pathology.   In general, staphylococci produce localized abscesses. It must be remembered, however, that the pathology also depends upon the route of introduction and the tissue involved. For example, if staphylococci are introduced upon the skin or mucous membrane, the resultant inflammation is usually chronic or mildly acute. On the other hand, if staphylococci are introduced beneath skin or mucous membranes, an acute process and abscess formation evolve. This is probably a result of the fact that the skin and mucous membranes are constantly inhabited by staphylococci and thereby develop a resistance to the organisms and possibly a partial immunity to pathogenic strains.

The discharge is usually purulent, even in mild infections of the mucous membranes. It may be abundant without much tissue· involvement. The bacteria proliferate upon the surface, usually without invading it. However, from any focus the staphylococcus may spread via the lymphatics and bloodstream, and venous thrombosis is a common finding. The organism is not found in living epithelium and is seldom phagocytized.

In the consideration of chronic recurrent staphylococcal infections, host resistance or hypersensitivity would seem even more important than bacterial virulence. Activation of susceptibility to staphylococci may be due to many factors: physical, including mascara, chemical, stress, poor sleep, pollution, and others.

Findings in the Eye.   Staphylococci are the most common, as well as the most thoroughly studied, cause of ocular infections. Staphylococci were once regarded simply as harmless conjunctival saprophytes. It is thus significant that experiments have established that ophthalmic staphylococci produce powerful toxins (Allen). The development of tests for pathogenicity is also of major importance (Suie and Taylor). With the advent of antibiotics we can now successfully treat *acute* staphylococcal infections, especially cellulitis, which were previously dangerous. However, treatment of *chronic* staphylococcal infections and prevention of their recurrence are still a serious problem in ophthalmology. The importance of allergic reactions to staphylococcal infections is now frequently discussed; all staphylococci may be antigenic. Unfortunately, allergy cannot be satisfactorily proven until the various types of sensitization are more fully understood (Theodore and Schlossman, 1958).

Two important factors that are not sufficiently stressed in the literature are (1) resistance of the body or local tissue, which in any chronic process is of primary importance, and (2) local ocular hygiene. It is known that, with low resistance, susceptibility is higher to any kind of stimulating or irritating factors, and the term "susceptibility" would appear preferable to "hypersensitivity."

Local hygiene of the eye can be remarkably effective without any other treatment. This includes removal of scales and crusts from lid margins (in blepharitis). Simply washing the face with hot water and mild soap, morning and night, can markedly improve the condition. Unfortunately, antibiotic ointment is often applied on top of heavy crusts.

Of all staphylococcal ocular diseases, blepharitis is the most common.

BLEPHARITIS. Two clinical forms are seen: ulcerative (Plate 1, Fig. 1) and squamous. Staphylococci (Plate 2, Fig. 6B) play a primary role in the ulcerative form and a secondary role in the squamous type, which is usually seborrheic, where the staphylococcus acts as a secondary invader. Either type may recur and persist for years. The condition is usually associated with conjunctivitis and purulent inflammation of the hair follicles as well as of the adjacent meibomian glands (hordeolum externum and internum). Accumulations of bacteria under the crusts of the ulcer or inside the meibomian glands (Scobee) result in a process of long duration and, often, hypersensitivity of tissue. Tylosis ciliaris (thickening of the lid margins) and madarosis (loss of cilia), caused by destruction of the hair follicles, are unpleasant complications of the process (Plate 2, Fig. 1). These irreversible changes are dangerous to the cornea because of exposure and dysfunction of the lacrimal film.

One of the causes of blepharoconjunctivitis is the pubic louse (Plate 39, Fig. 2A,B), which can be seen with the slit lamp when it attaches itself to the lashes. The adult louse is easily recognizable. The use of 0.25 percent physostygmine (eserine) ophthalmic ointment and mechanical removal will eliminate the parasite.

Pseudomonas blepharoconjunctivitis may develop on both lids as a result of myelosuppressive chemotherapy and is a very severe gangrenous disease.

CONJUNCTIVITIS. In adults, conjunctivitis is usually chronic and secondary to blepharitis. Involvement of the tarsal portion is pathognomonic for blepharitis, which is sometimes unnoticed, especially when mild. Chronic conjunctivitis (Thygeson et al) is most troublesome, particularly in old people, since it is of long duration and recurrent. In these cases, many other factors besides staphylococci have to be considered: dryness of the conjunctiva, wearing of contact lenses, use of mascara, metabolic disturbances, and others.

Acute conjunctivitis, seen usually in children, is less frequent than the chronic and may develop independently of blepharitis (Plate 1, Fig. 4). This has a rather typical appearance: (1) the lower palpebral conjunctiva predominantly is infected, (2) the discharge may be scanty or heavy, but the underlying tissue is little involved, (3) the condition is initially acute and if not properly treated may easily become chronic, and (4) corneal complications are not infrequent.

At this point, we must mention acute staphylococcal conjunctivitis of the newborn for this differs from the condition as manifested in later life. It is a purulent but superficial type with very little tissue involvement, probably due to prevention by coagulase action. Nevertheless, it can be as acute as gonococcal conjunctivitis. Corneal involvement is unknown, and there is no tendency to chronicity. The explanation of these peculiarities probably lies in some anatomic characteristics (absence of lymphatic tissue in the conjunctiva and rudimentary meibomian glands).

Phlyctenules are a frequent reaction to staphylococcal conjunctivitis, particularly in children. The lesions often ulcerate.

Children with lymphatic adenopathy often develop follicles, which may be numerous, predominantly in the lower fornix.

KERATITIS. Surprisingly, primary central staphylococcal hypopyon keratitis rarely results from corneal injury. The keratitis usually develops secondary to staphylococcal conjunctivitis or blepharoconjunctivitis.

The most frequent type of keratitis is marginal (Plate 1, Fig. 3), characterized by a small, grayish infiltrate adjacent to but often separated from the limbus by a narrow clear zone. The small, multiple infiltrates may run along the entire limbus. The infiltrated area ulcerates readily. The process may be caused by staphylococcal toxin, and bacteria are usually not found in the scraping from the ulcer. The keratitis is mild and is generally cured together with the conjunctivitis.

Superficial punctate keratitis also may complicate staphylococcal infection. Tiny punctate epithelial erosions, most marked in the lower half of the cornea, can be seen only by staining with fluorescein. This condition is most often observed in acute staphylococcal conjunctivitis, being probably an allergic reaction.

HORDEOLUM. Hordeolum internum is an acute inflammation of the meibomian glands, mainly caused by staphylococci (Plate 1, Fig. 2). The process is stubbornly resistant to treatment (drugs do not readily penetrate the glands). Hordeolum externum (acute inflammation of the Zeis glands) is also usually a staphylococcal infection. The process is more accessible to treatment. If it is localized at the angulus externus, a tremendous edema may develop, as the lymphatic ways cross here. *Hordeolosum*, the persistent recurrence of several hordeola, may be seen in patients with chronic blepharitis or conjunctivitis or in debilitated persons.

Staphylococci can also cause such dangerous diseases as orbital cellulitis and intraocular postoperative infection (Plate 2, Fig.6A). According to Allen, one-half of bacterial postoperative endophthalmitis is caused by staphylococci. In the majority of cases, it is a hospital-resistant strain (Burns). The lid margins and nasal passages are a potential source of infection. For diagnosis, the aspiration of the anterior chamber or vitreous is necessary. Unfortunately, diagnosis is not always successful, particularly after treatment.

Staphylococci are the most common secondary invaders in many conditions: dacryocystitis, trachoma, pemphigus, keratomalacia, and some others. In such viral infections as measles, influenza, and adenoviral infection, superimposed staphylococcal infection may have serious complications. Most frequently, staphylococcal infections of the eye are associated with skin diseases.

Treatment. Staphylococci are sensitive to sulfonamides and many other antibiotics, but their resistance to erythromycin and novobiocin may develop rapidly. The resistant strain often develops after prolonged use of antibiotics, particularly in chronic blepharoconjunctivitis. Treatment with the new antistaphylococcal drugs has to be restricted in routine diseases in order to preserve their value for serious infections. Therefore, sensitivity tests are necessary (Plate 2, Fig. 5) in all chronic and acute cases to insure the proper choice of antibiotics. Such therapy, to be successful, depends upon many additional factors. The medication should be discontinued if there is no response within a few days. Treatment with a particular antibiotic must immediately be stopped if sensitivity develops, and perhaps another used in its place.

While we must be concerned with proper treatment, it should be strongly emphasized that many cases are overtreated, and this may sometimes seriously complicate the picture.

Toxoid therapy should be tried in chronic recurrent infections if other therapy has failed (Julianelle et al; Thygeson, 1941). Staphylococcal antitoxin is of value only in cases of toxemia.

Regardless of the method of treatment, in blepharitis the lid margins must first be cleaned. The simplest method is to use hot compresses (with hot water or carbonate lotion or saline solution) for 5 to 10 minutes. The softened scales and crusts are then removed. Epilation of the lashes is indicated if there is suppuration of the hair follicles. Following these procedures, a variety of medications may be applied to the lids. Painting the lid margins with silver nitrate (1 percent or 2 percent) or with brilliant green (1 percent in 70 percent alcohol) is valuable in blepharitis.* Expressing the secretion from the meibomian glands and employing massage are highly recommended, especially in squamous blepharitis.

Attention to the health of the patient (good diet and hygiene—washing the face morning and night with hot water and mild soap) is helpful. Such predisposing factors as any kind of irritation must be considered.

The Streptococci

These are gram-positive cocci, typically arranged in chains. Streptococci cause a variety of severe diseases in man, among them scarlet fever, erysipelas, septicemia, infection of surgical wounds (sometimes fatal), cellulitis, puerperal fever, and epidemic sore throat. The incidence of streptococcal infection increases in the winter.

Streptococci also play an important role in various serious ocular infections, particularly cellulitis.

Allergy to streptococci or their products may be significant in rheumatic fever, nephritis, and endocarditis, and in such diseases of the eye as iridocyclitis.

There are a number of classifications of streptococci, two of which have received marked attention. Brown classified streptococci according to their action on blood agar. Of the streptococci to be discussed here, *Streptococcus pyogenes* shows beta hemolysis (complete), *Streptococcus mitis* shows alpha hemolysis (greenish, incomplete), and *Streptococcus salivarius* is nonhemolytic. Lancefield divided the streptococci into groups based on their antigenic properties.

Enterococci (*Streptococcus faecalis*) are a part of the normal flora of the intestinal tract. They may cause serious diseases, particularly in the urinary tract. Enterococci are resistant to many antimicrobial drugs, including penicillin.

Anaerobic streptococci were found recently to be a frequent cause of severe infection and gangrenous lesions (McEntyre, Ostler et al). They are often a part of the normal flora in the female genital tract.

We shall discuss the pathogenic strains as a whole.

Morphology. Streptococci are gram-positive, round or elongated cocci, usually flattened at adjacent sides. In smears from exudate or in fluid media, the organisms are typically arranged in long chains consisting of eight or more cocci, or in a diplococcal or occasionally rodlike

---

Apply brilliant green to the dried lid margin with a toothpick applicator, using a minimum amount of the stain.

form. However, extremely long chains may appear. On solid media, streptococci occur in pairs, short chains, or groups, closely resembling those of staphylococci (Plate 6, Fig. 4). The cocci vary greatly in size and in staining properties. In old cultures, club-shaped or gram-negative organisms may occur.

Encapsulation is not a typical characteristic of streptococci. When it does occur, it is more likely to be in members of Lancefield group A or in certain members of group C. The capsule lasts only for about the first two to two and a half hours of growth and disappears very quickly. There is probably no connection between encapsulation and virulence.

Culture. Streptococci require enriched media. On ordinary media, growth is poor. Blood agar plates are routinely used for primary isolation and determination of the type of hemolysis. The hemolysis is in an atmosphere of 10 percent carbon dioxide and influenced by the blood used. Horse or rabbit blood is best, and the medium should be glucose-free. On blood agar, colonies are pinpoint, grayish, and slightly opalescent, resembling small droplets of fluid and surrounded by a zone of hemolysis (incomplete in alpha, complete and sharply defined in beta). The minute colonies and large zone (2 to 4 mm) of hemolysis are important diagnostic characteristics (Plate 6, Fig. 3), although the size of the hemolytic zone varies considerably.

Depending upon the phase of dissociation, colonies may vary from the slimy mucoid types to granular or even dry.

Antigenic Structure. Many antigens have been isolated: group-specific carbohydrates, proteins, and nucleoproteins. Carbohydrates are contained in the cell wall of many streptococci, and these are the most important antigens for serologic grouping of streptococci.

Antigenic structures of hemolytic streptococci can be divided into serologic groups A to O (Lancefield). The majority of pathogenic streptococci fall into group A. Group C is important in neonatal sepsis and in meningitis. Serologic typing is more valuable than is hemolysis in the study of individual characteristics of streptococci. For practical reasons, however, identification according to type of hemolysis is still routine procedure in medical laboratories.

Among several antigenic substances is M protein, responsible for the virulence of group A streptococci, mainly by the prevention of phagocytosis. M protein also determines the type specificity of group A.

Pathogenicity. Pathogenicity is due to a variety of active substances, toxins and enzymes, elaborated by streptococci. Enzymes are the determining factors in pathogenicity, causing a marked invasiveness. They are as follows.

Streptokinase is an enzyme that dissolves human fibrin clots. Its action is indirect, but it is theorized that streptokinase activates plasminogen, which is a precursor of plasmin, a proteolytic ferment in plasma.

Streptodornase (deoxyribonuclease) lowers the viscosity of the exudate which has been caused by deoxyribonucleic acid (DNA). Streptodornase is closely related to streptococcal streptokinase. They have been employed clinically, individually or together, in a variety of conditions requiring enzymatic debridement. However, since both may be toxic, other enzymes, such as dornase, are preferred.

Hyaluronidase (spreading factor) splits hyaluronic acid, the substance cementing together connective tissue. Hyaluronidase is particularly responsible for diffusely spreading streptococcal infections and may facilitate the absorption and spread of injected drugs.

Hemolysins, streptolysins, leukocidins, and erythrogenic toxins are also responsible for pathogenicity. Erythrogenic toxin causes a rash in scarlet fever. The positive Dick test indicates susceptibility to erythrogenic toxin.

Pathology. In contrast to staphylococcal infections, streptococcal infections are serous or serosanguineous and usually not suppurative. The infection is generally diffuse and rapidly spreading, due to enzymes. The pyogenic process appears in the form of cellulitis rather than the localized abscess which is typical for staphylococcal infections.

Streptococcal diseases include general and local conditions, eg, general—acute and subacute endocarditis, local—sore throat, membranous conjunctivitis, corneal ulcer, impetigo (mainly in children and highly contagious). Local infections may become generalized and septicemic poststreptococcal diseases, eg, rheumatic fever and glomerular nephritis. Their latent period of one to four weeks suggests not the direct effect of bacteria but rather a hypersensitive response. In ophthalmology, uveitis belongs to this group.

Findings in the Eye. Cellulitis of the lid is most commonly caused by *S. pyogenes*. The eyebrow line is the usual site of infection. The process is generally associated with injury and may rarely follow metastasis of bacteria from distant parts of the body. It is characterized initially by localized infiltration and severe swelling. The process progresses rapidly, and massive necrosis may follow (Plate 6, Fig. 5). The infection may spread into the orbit or even into the brain or down the face.

Orbital cellulitis caused by *S. pyogenes,* prevalent in children, results chiefly from sinusitis or focal infections of the teeth or from pharyngitis. Panophthalmitis may ensue. The cellulitis may also be complicated by cavernous sinus thrombosis, which is always serious and can even be fatal.

Streptococcal panophthalmitis, postoperative or following injury, may occur (Plate 6, Fig. 6).

Lacrimal sac abscess due to streptococci, while uncommon, is sometimes seen. Very severe purulent keratitis may rarely develop (Plate 6, Fig. 2).

Streptococcal conjunctivitis with mild pseudomembrane formation or severe true membrane formation may develop. The latter is characterized by a coagulative fibrinous exudate, penetrating the epithelial and subepithelial tissues. The conjunctivitis is similar to that caused by *C. diphtheriae,* except that the bulbar as well as the palpebral conjunctiva is involved (Plate 6, Fig. 1). The process may be complicated by rapid necrosis of the cornea and perforation. Surprisingly, primary hypopyon keratitis due to *S. pyogenes* is rare (Vaughn). Streptococcal conjunctivitis of endogenous origin, which seldom occurs, is usually a mild pseudomembranous type which may persist for years or may recur. The conjunctival culture is usually negative.

Uveitis, iritis, and iridocyclitis, often resulting from streptococcal focal infections, are possibly allergic in nature.

In all of these severe ocular conditions, *Streptococcus pyogenes* is chiefly responsible. However, the role of *Streptococcus viridans* must be mentioned. Although the distinction between the hemolysis of alpha and beta streptococci is more quantitative than qualitative (Wilson and Miles), in practice this division is still recognized.

Streptococcus viridans (alpha) is not uncommonly a member of the normal flora. It can cause chronic focal infection and, in fact, does so more often than does *Streptococcus pyogenes.* As a result, *Streptococcus viridans* may be responsible for most streptococcal hypersensitivity. Serologically and biochemically, only a few strains of alpha streptococci are defined.

A great similarity in culture (Plate 5, Fig. 5) and appearance exists between *Streptococcus viridans* and the pneumococcus, except that the latter is encapsulated (Plate 5, Fig. 4A,B).

Both organisms produce similar eye infections, and both respond well to the same therapy. The infections are manifested as acute catarrhal conjunctivitis, hypopyon keratitis (Plate 5, Figs. 2, 3), chronic dacrocystitis, or postoperative infection (Plate 5, Fig. 1).

S. salivarius is usually considered nonpathogenic. Morphologically, it is similar to staphylococci or pathogenic streptococci. The most important identification is on the basis of cultural characteristics. *S. salivarius* grows luxuriantly on ordinary media and does not produce hemolysis.

The other streptococci, such as enterococci, are frequently the cause of urinary tract infections but rarely of ocular diseases (Spaeth).

The source of pathogenic streptococci is man, who distributes the organism to others via droplets on the skin.

Treatment. Practically all streptococci are susceptible to sulfonamides and penicillin, and most of them are susceptible to erythromycin. Some are resistant to tetracycline. Alpha streptococci and enterococci vary in their antibiotic sensitivity, and tests for such sensitivity are essential. No significant resistance of streptococci to penicillin is yet known. Sulfadiazine has been found highly effective in group A hemolytic streptococcal infections. However, exquisite sensitivity of a host to penicillin is not uncommon. Consequently, care must be taken when penicillin is given by parenteral injection.

The Pneumococcus *(Streptococcus pneumoniae)*

The pneumococcus, formerly *Diplococcus pneumoniae,* has been reclassified as *Streptococcus pneumoniae* in the 8th edition of *Bergey's Manual of Determinative Bacteriology.* Pneumococci are common inhabitants of the upper respiratory tract and are the primary cause of over 80 percent of lobar pneumonia cases. The organisms were recognized by Pasteur in 1881, and in 1886 Frankel and Weichselbaum described the pneumococcus as the agent of pneumonia. Before sulfonamides and antibiotics, the mortality from pneumococcal pneumonia was high, particularly in infants and the aged.

Various studies have indicated that *S. pneumoniae* occurs frequently (40 to 70 percent) in the normal conjunctival flora and nasolacrimal system.

S. pneumoniae causes severe and serious ocular diseases (Okumoto et al). Because pneumococci are often present in normal flora, any ocular injury may lead to severe purulent infection, the most frequent being a hypopyon keratitis.

Morphology. The organisms are gram-positive, lancet-shaped, and occur in pairs. The diplococcal arrangement is found in clinical material (Plate 3, Fig. 5) and in smears from colonies grown on solid media. In fluid media, the cells occur chiefly in short chains (in contrast to the long chains of other streptococci) (Plate 4, Fig. 2). Pneumococci can be decolorized very easily, showing some gram-negative forms, particularly in aged or very young cultures. The majority of pneumococci possess a polysaccharide capsule (Plate 4, Fig. 1). This results in the appearance of smooth colonies. However, in any culture of pneumococci, a few nonencapsulated variants may occur, giving rise to rough colonies. This may be associated with drug resistance.

Culture. The pneumococcus does not grow on the usual media but requires an enriched medium.

On blood agar plates, in a candle jar, almost all ophthalmologic pneumococci appear as small, flat in the center with elevated rim, shiny colonies surrounded by a green zone of incomplete alpha hemolysis (Plate 4, Fig. 4). The easily recognized green appearance is the most characteristic feature.

Differential diagnosis between pneumococci and other alpha streptococci can be made as follows: pneumococci are usually encapsulated, whereas other alpha streptococci are nonencapsulated. The bile solubility test, optochin sensitivity test (Plate 4, Figs. 3,5), and inulin fermentation are positive for pneumococci, negative for other alpha streptococci.

Antigenic Structure. Cooper and other workers identified 32 serologic types of pneumococci; at present, there are known to be at least 80 or more. Types I to VIII are responsible for most pneumococcal diseases. In ocular diseases, types I, II, and III are most common. For serologic differentiation two components are important. One is a polysaccharide SSS (specific soluble substance) present in the capsular material. Capsular polysaccharides determine both virulence and type of pneumococcus. It has been shown that antibodies against the pneumococcus are induced by capsular material and are type-specific. The other is protein M (group-specific) found in the somatic portion of the pneumococcus.

Immunity to pneumococcal infection is unfortunately incomplete and of brief duration only.

PNEUMOCOCCUS TYPING. When pneumococci are mixed with type-specific rabbit antiserum, swelling of the capsule develops (Neufeld or Quellung reaction). The technique is simple: a loopful of undiluted antiserum is mixed with the specimen on the slide and covered. Then a loopful of Löffler's alkaline methylene blue is added at the margin of the coverglass. The capsule can also be demonstrated by the Hiss copper sulfate method of staining* (Plate 4, Fig. 1).

Capsule Stain (Hiss Method)
   Materials:
1.   Gentian violet or fuchsin solution
     Saturated alcoholic solution of
          gentian violet or basic fuchsin   5 ml
     Distilled water   95 ml
2.   Copper sulfate
     Copper sulfate   20 ml
     Water   100 ml

Intraperitoneal inoculation of white mice is the most rapid method of obtaining a pure culture of pneumococci from contaminated material. It also determines the pathogenicity and demonstrates the capsule.

Pathogenicity and Pathology. Pneumococci do not produce toxins. However, there is some evidence of their toxic ability, which may possibly play a role in the extensive destruction of tissue in corneal hypopyon ulcer (Johnson and Allen, 1971, 1975). The disease process is mainly caused by the invasiveness and multiplication of the bacteria. The capsular polysaccharides are the determining factor in the virulence of the pneumococci and in the development of the disease. In addition, the capsule itself delays or prevents ingestion of pneumococci by phagocytosis. Predisposing factors, such as intercurrent infections, viral infections, sickle cell anemia, alcoholic intoxication, debility, and many others, are sometimes more important in the development of pneumococcal infection than is the virulence of the agent.

The characteristic pathology of pneumococcal infections is marked edema and fibrinous exudate. Both the onset and determination of the infection are sudden. The role of allergy in pneumococcal infection has been neglected. The sudden explosive onset of pneumococcal infection suggests an allergic reaction in individuals previously having pneumococcal infection. It occurs more often in adults than in children. Allergic reactions of the urticarial type may occur when convalescence begins.

Pneumococci also cause sinusitis and otitis which may, by dissemination, cause meningitis and endocarditis.

Pneumococcal infection is usually endemic, and carriers are responsible for spreading the infection.

Resistance. Pneumococci are delicate organisms which die rapidly. They are readily killed by heat, with death occurring after only 10 minutes at 52 C. However, they often survive well at low temperatures, even at the freezing point.

Findings in the Eye. The pneumococcus may cause a destructive hypopyon keratitis, is often found in chronic dacryocystitis, and is a frequent cause of acute conjunctivitis. It does not ordinarily cause chronic conjunctivitis or blepharoconjunctivitis.

CONJUNCTIVITIS. Epidemics of acute pneumococcal conjunctivitis have been described, and it is the most common type in many parts of the United States. The infection seems to be more prevalent in the

---

The best source of material for the demonstration of capsules by this method is infected exudate from the animal body. If a stock culture is to be examined, the organisms should be emulsified in a drop of serum on the slide.

Technic:
1. The film is dried but not fixed with heat.
2. Flood the glass slide with gentian violet or fuchsin solution.
3. Hold the preparation for a second over a free flame until it steams.
4. Wash off the dye with the copper sulfate solution (do not wash with water).
5. Blot.

colder months and in northern climates. Frequent association with a cold in the head (but not with pneumonia) is characteristic. The infection has a predilection for children. Pneumococcal conjunctivitis, similar to the conjunctivitis caused by the Koch-Weeks bacillus, is usually of moderate severity with a mild mucopurulent exudation. However, pronounced redness of the bulbar conjunctiva, often associated with petechial hemorrhages, is seen, usually in the upper fornix (Plate 3, Fig. 1). These are more marked in pneumococcal conjunctivitis than in that due to the Koch-Weeks bacillus and are probably bacterial allergic reactions. Chemosis of the bulbar conjunctiva and enlargement of the preauricular glands may occur in severe cases.

Follicle formation is not infrequent in children but is quite rare in pneumococcal conjunctivitis of adults.

It should be pointed out that the clinical appearance of pneumococcal conjunctivitis seems to vary in different countries. The discharge may become abundant and purulent, and corneal involvement is frequent. This picture is also seen in mixed infection, particularly with staphylococci.

The disease is contagious, and in smear numerous typical diplococci are usually seen. The exudate smear may be sufficient for diagnosis (Plate 3, Fig. 5). The pneumococci disappear rapidly in the regressive stage and are replaced by *Corynebacterium xerosis* and staphylococci. Subsidence of the conjunctivitis, even without treatment, is characteristic and occurs rapidly.

Corneal complications are rare in the United States. If they do occur, they are usually in the form of marginal infiltrates which later break down, forming small ulcers. The condition is not severe and heals along with the conjunctivitis. During the conjunctivitis, a few punctate, staining lesions may be seen in the epithelial layer of the cornea.

PNEUMOCOCCAL ULCER (ULCUS SERPENS).   The pneumococcus is the commonest cause of central corneal ulcer (Rhodes; Vaughn), particularly in countries where chronic infection of the nasal mucosa is frequent. This results in blockage of the lacrimal passage, and the lacrimal sac serves as a main reservoir for pneumococcal infection. It is more common among farmers, stonemasons, coal miners, or debilitated persons. Pneumococci do not invade normal corneal epithelium. The portal of entry is usually through a corneal abrasion, generally caused by a foreign body.

This pneumococcal corneal ulcer is central and usually occurs as a primary entity without a preceding conjunctivitis. The ulcer is typically associated with sterile hypopyon. The hypopyon indicates an iritis or iridocyclitis due to toxic products. If the cornea is perforated, an infected hypopyon is likely. The clinical picture is characterized initially by a heavy infiltrate, yellowish in color, which rapidly breaks down, resulting in ulcer formation. The ulcer spreads on the surface of the cornea in a particular direction, hence the name "serpiginous ulcer" or "ulcus serpens" of Saemisch (1870) is used (Duke-Elder, p. 1934). The spreading, or progressive, margin is usually undermined in pocketlike formation (Plate 3, Fig. 2). The organisms are numerous there, and the scraping should be taken from this area. The typical morphology of pneumococci may be sufficient to be diagnostic in the scraping. Later, the ulceration extends more deeply, and perforation of the cornea often follows. Then the infection may become intraocular or even result in panophthalmitis.

Pneumococci are still regarded by many authorities as the principal etiologic agent for central hypopyon ulcer.

Some metastatic pneumococcal eye infections have been recorded recently: two cases of endophthalmitis in multiple myeloma (Baker and Spencer) and a hypopyon (Macoul).

CHRONIC DACRYOCYSTITIS.   This almost always arises secondarily to obstruction or stenosis of the nasolacrimal duct. When free drainage through the duct is hindered, stasis of tears results, and this is a favorable condition for infection. In the warm, dark lacrimal sac with its sufficient food, the bacteria grow as in an incubator. A large number of encapsulated pneumococci are most commonly found within it, along with other organisms. A lacrimal sac so affected becomes a constant source of infection for the eye, and while always dangerous, it is even more so when overlooked before intraocular surgery. Chronic dacryocystitis can easily be missed because there is little or no local inflammation. This has been called by Theodore (1948) "silent" dacryocystitis. In cases of chronic unilateral conjunctivitis, chronic dacryocystitis must be first suggested. Examination of the nasolacrimal system before intraocular surgery is recommended, especially for older patients. The examination should include pressure over the lacrimal sac as well as irrigation.

The chronic process may suddenly exacerbate into acute dacryocystitis if the infection invades the perilacrimal tissue. Many factors, often unrecognizable, may play a role. If a lacrimal fistula develops (Plate 3, Fig. 4) and is long existing, granulomatous masses resembling tumor may result (Plate 3, Fig. 3).

Postoperative infections are often caused by pneumococci, and this organism is by far the most common pathogen for panophthalmitis following wounds of the eye.

Bacterial metastasis in pneumococcal septicemia has been found in the form of small, translucent nodules in the choroid or retina.

Treatment.   Before the antibiotic era, optochin (ethyl-hydrocuprein hydrochloride) was regarded as specific treatment for pneumococcal infection. It can be given only locally, as it is highly toxic systemically. In superficial infections such as conjunctivitis, 1 percent optochin solution is useful, especially in areas where antibiotics are difficult to obtain.

The pneumococcus is sensitive to most antibiotics and sulfonamides, giving rapid recovery. Penicillin is the drug of choice, but a significant resistance to it and to tetracycline and neomycin has been noted recently. Since there may be a recurrence, continuation of treatment for one week after the disappearance of clinical symptoms is recommended.

Antibiotics can be applied locally or systemically. In conjunctivitis, local therapy suffices. In cases of hypopyon ulcer both local and systemic administration of antibiotics is required. For the latter, the usual treatment is from 300,000 to 1 million units of penicillin three times a day.

If dacryocystitis is present, dacryocystectomy should be considered. Most attempts to treat central hypopyon ulcer in the presence of dacryocystitis have proved unsuccessful.

Proper care of the iris must not be forgotten.

THE *CORYNEBACTERIUM* GENUS

As the name implies, corynebacteria are clublike in form, because of the presence of Babes-Ernst metachromatic granules.

Included in this genus are the broad group of diphtheroids and *Corynebacterium diphtheriae*. Most diphtheroids are human parasites, living mainly on the skin and mucous membranes. *C. xerosis* is an almost constant saprophyte of the conjunctiva. While saprophytic for man, some diphtheroids are pathogenic for animals.

Of the entire group, only *C. diphtheriae* (the diphtheria bacillus) is an important human pathogen.

Corynebacterium diphtheriae

While no longer a serious problem in many areas, diphtheria was formerly a dread disease. Even today in areas where immunization is not practical, the infection is still a severe threat, especially for children.

Morphology.   While this bacillus is gram-positive, the gram stain is of little value in studying its morphology. To demonstrate the metachromatic granules, a special stain, such as Neisser's,* must be used. Methylene blue is a good routine diagnostic stain. Diphtheria bacilli are large and slender, straight or slightly curved, pleomorphic rods (Plate 8, Fig. 3). The metachromatic granules are typically situated at the poles, the rod being a drumstick shape. The bacilli are arranged at various angles to one another, forming V, T, or L shapes, and groups of the organisms form clusters resembling Chinese letters. This appearance aids considerably in diagnosis. In smear from the culture, true branching may be seen.

C. diphtheriae is divided into three subgroups: gravis, mitis, and intermedius, depending upon the grade of infectivity. The subgroups have much in common.

Culture. Diphtheria bacilli grow slowly on ordinary media. The best medium is Löffler's blood serum medium. Use of a routine blood agar plate is advisable for identification of other bacteria, especially hemolytic streptococci, which may occur together with C. diphtheriae.

Colonies of C. diphtheriae on Löffler's medium are small, round, granular, moist, slightly creamy or gray, and have irregular edges (Plate 8, Fig. 5). Tellurite medium is used in addition to Löffler's blood serum medium to differentiate C. diphtheriae from the diphtheroid bacilli and to distinguish subgroups of C. diphtheriae (gravis, mitis, and intermedius). The colonies of C. diphtheriae are a distinct black due to reduction of tellurite (Plate 8, Fig. 4A).

On blood agar, colonies are usually small, grayish, and granular. Beta hemolysis may be slight or absent (Plate 8, Fig. 4B).

In contrast to the slowly growing diphtheroids, the diphtheria bacilli grow rapidly, requiring only 6 to 12 hours of incubation.

In its biochemical reactions, C. diphtheriae produces acid (not gas) in glucose but not in sucrose (Plate 9, Fig. 4).

*Neisser Stain
1. Methylene blue (Neisser s)

Methylene blue	1 g
Alcohol, 96 percent	20 ml
Glacial acetic acid	50 ml
Water	950 ml

2. Bismarck brown

Bismarck brown	1 g
Water	100 ml

For staining Klebs-Loffler bacilli and C. xerosis to show metachromatic granules. Use a 24 hour culture on blood serum. Make films and stain with methylene blue for one-half minute. Wash in tap water and treat with Bismarck brown for one-half minute. Wash, dry, and mount. The metachromatic granules stain very dark; the bodies light yellow.

Toxin Production and Pathogenicity.   C. *diphtheriae* produces a powerful exotoxin, is not invasive, and the bacteria hardly ever enter the bloodstream. The toxin is the principal factor in establishing disease. It rapidly diffuses from the primary focus, chiefly tonsillitis, to other parts of the body, and toxemia may result.

The toxin stimulates formation of a powerful antitoxin, which imparts prolonged immunity. Antiserum containing powerful antibodies, important for treatment, is prepared by repeated injection of purified toxoid into various animals, such as rabbits, guinea pigs, horses, and sheep.

Pathology.   Diphtheria bacilli cause a local infection of the mucous membranes, particularly the pharynx and more rarely the conjunctiva. The epithelium becomes necrotic from absorbed toxin and is embedded in a massive fibropurulent exudate, forming a pseudomembrane. If subepithelial tissue is involved, a true membrane develops. The capillaries enter the membrane, and therefore bleeding occurs if one attempts to remove it. The bacilli multiply in this tissue, and their toxin is rapidly absorbed. It may damage distant parts of the body, causing parenchymatous degeneration, fatty infiltration, necrosis, or gross hemorrhages. The toxin often damages the nerves, resulting in paralysis, and the eye may be involved.

Findings in the Eye.   C. *diphtheriae* is a cause of conjunctivitis, although this is now rare. Depending upon the severity of the process, two clinical types of conjunctivitis are distinguished: pseudomembranous and true membranous. Both usually follow pharyngeal diphtheria in children aged 2 to 8. The pseudomembrane may be removed without resultant bleeding, whereas removal of a true membrane leads to bleeding. In the latter, the entire conjunctival tissue to the tarsal plate may be penetrated by a thick network of fibrin (Plate 8, Fig. 1) and the vessels obliterated by thrombosis.

Three stages are characteristic in severe membranous conjunctivitis.

1. Infiltrated or indurated stage: the lids and conjunctiva become almost impossible to evert. Pressure from the tense indurated lids may cause corneal damage, even necrosis.
2. Suppurative stage: the lids soften, the membrane separates, and underlying granulation may be seen.
3. Cicatrization stage: scarring of the lid conjunctiva is seen.

Diphtheritic infections may be complicated by other bacterial invaders, including staphylococci, pneumococci, and streptococci. The latter severely aggravate the process.

The *C. diphtheriae* cells usually disappear by the time the membrane is gone, but some persons become chronic carriers.

Diphtheritic mucopurulent conjunctivitis, indistinguishable from other bacterial conjunctivitides, may also be seen (Plate 8, Fig. 2). Conjunctivitis due to *C. diphtheriae* is rare in the United States, and when it occurs, it is almost always the pseudomembranous type. It is rarely associated with pharyngeal diphtheria, and there may or may not be systemic symptoms. Active immunization of children by diphtheria toxoid is not permanent; hence the disease may occur in previously immunized adults.

Before the introduction of active immunization, diphtheria was a disease attacking small children. It now occurs in adult life, often in epidemic proportions. It is evident that this immunization is not long-lasting and infection can recur without a booster (Joklik W, Willet G). Before the immunization era, subclinical infection was common, which stimulated antibody production to a high level. In addition there were carriers, who helped in the production of antibodies. Both are now lacking.

Corneal involvement may be due directly to toxin, to lid pressure as mentioned before, and to the decrease of corneal nutrition resulting from thrombosis of limbal capillaries. The typically necrotic diphtheritic keratitis may become purulent because of secondary infection. Ulceration and perforation of the cornea may result.

Palsy of extraocular muscles or, more frequently, paralysis of accommodation may occur. The latter is usually permanent.

Diagnosis. There are no differential diagnostic indications in the clinical picture of conjunctivitis. Diagnosis depends almost entirely on bacteriologic examination, a problem involving delay. The bacteriologist with long experience may obtain a rapid preliminary diagnosis by direct, specially stained smears. Otherwise, the diagnosis requires several days of special study. This must be confirmed by cultural identification of the organism and by the virulence test.

VIRULENCE TEST. The most definitive type of testing is by intracutaneous or cutaneous inoculation of a bacterial suspension into guinea pigs or rabbits. This test is not practical from a clinical standpoint, as it takes much time and is quite costly. For these reasons, the in vitro test is recommended (Plate 9, Fig. 2).

In vitro test (Jawetz et al 1970, p 184):

A strip of filter paper, saturated with antitoxin, is placed on an agar plate containing 20 percent horse serum. The cultures to be tested for toxigenicity are streaked across the plate at right angles to the filter paper. After 48 hours incubation, the antitoxin diffusion from the paper strip has precipitated the toxin diffusion from the toxigenic cultures in lines radiating from the intersection of the streak of bacterial growth.

This test is best done in a general bacteriology laboratory. If the ophthalmologist suspects diphtheria, he should immediately send test material to the bacteriology laboratory.

Treatment.   Antidiphtheritic serum therapy is specific. Antitoxin should be given as soon as the diagnosis is made. In severe cases, intravenous injection of large doses (4,000 or 6,000 or 10,000 units) is necessary. Usually one injection is enough, but if necessary it can be repeated in 10 to 12 hours to avoid anaphylactic reaction. In mild cases 2,000 units intramuscularly may be satisfactory. Antibiotics topically and warm compresses are required. If membranes are present, avoid the use of silver nitrate. To prevent secondary infection, such antibiotics as penicillin, streptomycin, tetracycline, or erythromycin may be needed.

Corynebacterium xerosis

C. *xerosis* alone of the numerous diphtheroids (Chase et al) is considered a strictly ophthalmic bacterium. It has not been found on any other organ than the conjunctiva, and it is almost constantly present there. It grows as a saprophyte, usually on desquamating conjunctival epithelium. This bacillus has never been shown to be pathogenic for the eye. However, its pathogenicity has been shown in experiments (Weiss et al). It should not be forgotten that some diphtheroids can be pathogenic for animals. C. *xerosis* often confuses laboratory diagnosis because of morphologic characteristics similar to those of other bacteria.

Morphology.   The bacilli are short, thick, curved, and grampositive, with very irregular size and shape. Metachromatic granules are generally distributed throughout the whole bacillus, giving it a barred appearance (Plate 7, Figs. 2, 6). The organisms are frequently seen in clumps or arranged at angles giving V, L, and T formations, or in palisades. In smear, C. *xerosis* may be confused with the pneumococcus if the metachromatic granules are isolated at the poles, thus giving intensive bipolar staining. At other times, the bacillus may have a beaded form and thus be confused with streptococci. Most important for the identification of this organism is the irregularity of its size and shape, and even when there are V or L forms, one bacillus tends to be of different size and shape from the other (Plate 7, Figs. 1, 2).

C. *xerosis* differs from C. *diphtheriae* by being shorter, thicker, and more clumped and curved. Usually the metachromatic granules are not at the end of the organism but are distributed throughout its whole body (Plate 9, Fig. 1).

Culture. C. *xerosis* grows much more slowly than does C. *diphtheriae,* sometimes taking a few days to a week, averaging 48 hours. Colonies on blood agar (Plate 9, Fig. 3) are tiny, dustlike, gray, opaque, dull, and dry looking (Plate 7, Figs. 5A, B). They adhere firmly to the medium and do not emulsify easily. On Löffler's serum (Plate 9, Fig. 3), they grow faster, though not as quickly as C. *diphtheriae,* and the colonies are smaller and drier.

C. *xerosis* produces acid in glucose and sucrose.

Findings in the Eye. C. *xerosis* is not a pathogen but rather a normal inhabitant of the conjunctiva. The bacilli may appear in large numbers in any infectious conjunctivitis, especially during the period of convalescence: In some infections they are present throughout the course, because of a symbiotic relationship with etiologic bacteria, such as *Moraxella* organisms. A large number of C. *xerosis* cells may be found in vitamin A deficiency because of the marked keratinization of the conjunctival epithelium (Tourean et al). Scraping from Bitot's spot (Plate 7, Figs. 1, 3) shows the amount of the organisms to be similar to that in a smear from pure culture. An increased amount of C. *xerosis* may indicate any dry condition of the eye.

A large number of cells of C. *xerosis* are invariably present in keratomalacia (Baum et al). This condition, with complete destruction of the cornea, occurs usually in children who are debilitated and malnourished (Plate 7, Fig. 4).

AEROBIC SPOREFORMING BACILLI

To this group belong a large number of saprophytic strains, including *Bacillus cereus* and *Bacillus subtilis* (Plate 9, Fig. 5) (Davenport). They are inhabitants of soil, water, air, and vegetation. *Bacillus anthracis* is the only species of this genus pathogenic for man.

Bacillus anthracis

Anthrax was known even in antiquity. It was the first disease of proven bacterial origin. The disease is still widespread, occurring in every country, although it is prevalent only in certain areas. In the United States about 50 cases of anthrax are reported every year.

Morphology. These bacilli are large, square-ended, gram-positive organisms, usually arranged in long chains. Their spores are situated at about the center of the organism. The bacilli are nonmotile. Culture of the patient's blood or a specimen from the lesion or both are necessary for diagnosis of infection.

Cultivation. B. anthracis is aerobic (or facultatively anaerobic) and grows well on nutrient agar and other general media. Blood agar is used to differentiate the usually nonhemolytic B. anthracis from the known hemolytic, saprophytic strains of the species. However, the test for pathogenicity is essential. The colonies appear round, with a cut-glass appearance. The membranous consistency of the colonies is due to the formation of parallel chains by the bacilli.

Pathogenicity and Pathology. B. anthracis is pathogenic for man and most animals. Grazing animals, such as sheep and cattle, are more commonly affected. Man may be infected by the wool (woolsorter's disease), hair, or hide of diseased animals. Anthrax is primarily a disease of the skin, affecting especially such exposed areas as the head and neck. Infection follows injury to the skin. The bacilli spread via lymphatics to the bloodstream and multiply rapidly (Krauss and Spikes). Bacilli are easily demonstrated at the ulcerative stage. If untreated, the disease is usually followed by septicemia and death. The organism proliferates at the site of entry, and the disease is established primarily by the invasion and multiplication of bacilli.

Findings in the Eye. Anthrax of the lid occurs but is extremely rare. The manifestations are similar to anthrax infections of other parts of the body. Two clinical forms occur: (1) malignant pustule and (2) malignant edema. The site of a malignant pustule can be on either lid. It begins in the form of a pimple, followed by a vesicle, then by a pustule, and finally an ulcer or gangrene. The lesion is not painful, and the regional lymph glands are only mildly involved. Large areas may be involved, and heavy scarring is a sequela. The process may extend to involve the cornea and other parts of the eye. Ulceration of the cornea, panophthalmitis, and exophthalmos with optic atrophy may occur.

Malignant edema of the lid is characterized by marked edema, with the skin showing little or no inflammation. These cases are more difficult to diagnose, and septicemia is more likely to occur in this form of anthrax.

Treatment. Most antibiotics are effective against anthrax bacilli. Treatment must be started early to prevent development of a toxic process. Antisera and antibiotics considerably reduce mortality. To prevent the spread of infection, control measures and active immunization of domestic animals and anyone having had contact with infection are mandatory.

ANAEROBIC SPORE-FORMING BACILLI

The Clostridia

Except for *Clostridium* bacilli, anaerobes have generally been dismissed as harmless saprophytes. Only recently have anaerobes, eg, various anaerobic streptococci, been recognized as a major cause of serious infection. *Bacteroides fragilis* arose as the most common pathogen and is often not sensitive to penicillin.

A number of species belong to the genus *Clostridium*. They are distributed in soil or in the intestinal tract of both man and animals. They become pathogenic in injured tissue, producing toxin and rapid putrefaction of protein. The most common pathogenic strains for man are *Clostridium botulinum, Clostridium tetani,* and *Clostridium perfringens.*

Morphologically, clostridia are gram-positive, with a drumstick appearance. Bulging of the wall at one end of the rod is caused by spores. While the arrangement of the organism varies, it is often seen in long chains. Meticulous collection of specimens and a special culture technique are required. Even brief exposure to air can kill the bacteria. The cultivation period in Brewer's thioglycollate broth is about 10 days, but cultivation is difficult, since the bacilli of this genus are strictly anaerobic. It is best to have these specimens examined by a general bacteriologist if no properly equipped laboratory is available.

C. botulinum causes intoxication by the ingestion of infected food (eg, smoked, home-canned, and unboiled food). Eye findings (König, Tsutsui) are secondary to systemic symptoms and include incoordination of eye muscles, double vision, and paralysis. Treatment is principally by administration of polyvalent antitoxin. Laboratory diagnosis is based on the demonstration of toxin in leftover food, since culture is usually useless.

C. tetani produces toxemia and is not an invasive organism. Infection remains strictly localized in the area of devitalized tissue (wounds, burn injuries, surgical sutures). The toxin damages the nervous system, resulting in muscle spasm. Nearly three-quarters of known cases of tetanus over a 10-year period in New York occurred in narcotics addicts, with high mortality rate.

C. perfringens produces about 12 toxins, including alpha toxin, lecithinase, the most potent of them all. This is hemolytic, necrotizing, and lethal. The infection remains localized, while the toxin and tissue necrosis involve systemic reactions. The biochemical alteration in the presence of a lowered oxidation-reduction potential is of primary importance, and there are other significant factors, such as damage to vessels, the presence of necrotizing tissue, and the utilization of oxygen by bacteria. Gas gangrene, a wartime wound infection, is caused by *C. perfringens*. It is difficult to establish its etiologic role in wounds or in panophthalmitis, since clostridia are mixed with many other cocci and bacilli.

C. *perfringens* occurs in the female genitourinary tract as part of the normal flora. It can cause infection following the use of instruments in abortion.

Ocular infection caused by this species is relatively rare, and the literature on this subject is limited. Gas gangrene of the lids or orbit may develop following injury and then contact with contaminated soil or manure. C. *perfringens*, if introduced into the eye through a wound, including postoperative wounds, may cause severe panophthalmitis. Fifty-nine or more cases of gas gangrene panophthalmitis are recorded (McEntyre, Curran and Leavelle). This is characterized by a bubble in the anterior chamber and a brownish exudate. In our experience, panophthalmitis with bubbles in the anterior chamber and cornea were found in a case of *Escherichia coli* infection. Corneal ulcers have been reported, with total edema and a bubble in the superior layers. Conjunctivitis involving the lower fornix with multiple hemorrhages is also known (Henkind and Fedukowicz). A violent infection often associated with other organisms, especially streptococci, may occur. Except for gas gangrene, other clostridial eye infections are only secondary to systemic diseases.

Treatment. Since in clostridial infections toxin is the factor establishing the process, antitoxin must be used in treatment. It is usually polyvalent, containing antibodies to several toxins, and it should be administered as soon as possible. The antitoxin can be used together with antibiotics.

THE MYCOBACTERIA

This group is comprised of acid-fast bacilli, the majority of which are saprophytic. *Mycobacterium tuberculosis*, *Mycobacterium bovis*, and *Mycobacterium leprae* are known pathogens for man. They are intracellular parasites which usually cause a chronic granulomatous process.

Mycobacterium tuberculosis and *Mycobacterium bovis*

M. *tuberculosis* and M. *bovis* are equally pathogenic for man by either the respiratory or the gastrointestinal route. The more common is M. *tuberculosis*, which invades the body by being inhaled or ingested, or directly through the skin or mucous membranes.

The location and pattern of the tuberculous lesions indicate the route of primary infection. If invasion is by inhalation, tuberculosis of the lungs develops. Scrofula or cervical adenitis results from ingestion. Entrance through the skin or mucous membranes is usually followed by arid ulcers, with marked enlargement of the regional lymph nodes. An example is oculoglandular Parinaud's syndrome in primary tuberculosis of the conjunctiva.

Morphology.   In smear, the acid-fast tubercle bacilli are fairly long, straight, curved, or bent. With Ziehl-Neelsen stain (see Chapter 5) they appear irregularly red with a granular or beaded appearance. They may occur singly or in groups. If the organisms are arranged at angles to each other, they resemble corynebacteria. Their appearances are so characteristic that identification can usually be made by microscopic examination of a direct smear (Plate 10, Fig. 4).

In animal tissue, the bacilli are more regular, longer, and thinner. In culture, there is pleomorphism, with coccoid, club-shaped, filamentous, or even branching forms.

Tubercle bacilli take the gram stain poorly and hence are not classified by this method but rather by acid-fast staining. The simplest and most commonly used stain is Ziehl-Neelsen's. Numerous other staining methods, including fluorescent microscopy, have been utilized.

Culture.   Cultivation of tubercle bacilli is a difficult and prolonged procedure. They are strictly aerobic (probably the chief basis for the success of lung collapse therapy). A variety of complicated media have been used to grow the bacilli, which grow best on media enriched with egg yolk. On Löwenstein's medium, satisfactory for both *M. tuberculosis* and *M. bovis* (Plate 10, Fig. 5), the colonies are creamy, dull, rough, and granular. Growth requires at least two months.

Chemical Composition.   Tubercle bacilli contain high percentages of lipids which are possibly responsible for cellular reaction and granulation. Proteins (largely nucleoproteins) are responsible for tuberculin sensitivity and stimulation of antibody production. The bacilli also contain a relatively small amount of polysaccharides, which possibly can induce an anaphylactic type of hypersensitivity.

Pathology.   Primary and reactivating tuberculosis are distinguishable. Primary Ghon complex develops at the base of the lung and is associated with lymph node involvement.

The reactivating type can be of endogenous origin, caused by surviving bacteria or from the surrounding environment. This is a more chronic process of the productive type (granuloma, tubercle), usually located at the apex. Lymph nodes may be only slightly involved.

The pathology is determined by the virulence and number of tubercle bacilli and, more important, the resistance and hypersensitivity of the host. Two types of lesions are produced. One is the exudative acute inflammatory type (Plate 10, Fig.3), which can either be absorbed or result in massive necrosis and ulceration. This process in the lungs is similar to bacterial pneumonia. The other is a productive type characterized by a chronic granuloma or tubercle. The tubercle consists of a central zone in which are found typical Langhans' giant cells and mononuclear epithelioid cells. The central zone is surrounded by a cuff of lymphocytes. Dead tissue at the center of the tubercle becomes cheesy (caseated); this may be followed by a cavity or fibrosis and calcification. The tubercle bacilli are found intracellularly in monocytes, giant cells, or reticuloendothelial cells. The bacilli may spread from the initial site via lymphatics and the bloodstream to all organs, causing miliary tuberculosis. (If the spread is via lymphatics, the regional glands are first involved.)

Tuberculin Diagnostic Methods. Tuberculin is an extract of tubercle bacilli or a filtrate of a broth culture. Koch, using tuberculin for subcutaneous injections, produced a local inflammation in tuberculous animals, followed by necrosis. This has since been known as "Koch's phenomenon," a state of hypersensitivity induced by previous exposure to tubercle bacilli. The reaction is negative in normal animals. Hence, Koch's phenomenon is an important diagnostic indication.

There are now available various kinds of tuberculin for diagnostic or therapeutic purposes. The best known are Koch's original tuberculin, known as Old Tuberculin (OT), and Seibert's purified protein derivative (PPD), which is preferable.

Several tuberculin diagnostic tests have been devised: the Mantoux intracutaneous test, the Pirquet cutaneous test, and the Vollmer patch test. The Mantoux test is the most popular because it is the most accurate and gives quantitative measurement. Koch's original subcutaneous injection is now used only in veterinary practice.

Some individuals, particularly Blacks or patients with tuberculous eye diseases, may be extremely sensitive to tuberculin. Therefore, an initial dose must be given with caution, since it can activate primary silent lesions.

The tuberculin tests are of value in young children, although a positive test does not indicate present, active disease, only past infection. It may be negative if the tuberculous infection is superimposed by measles or Boeck's sarcoid, in anergy, in immunosuppressive drug therapy, or under other circumstances.

The diagnosis is established only by the finding of tubercle bacilli.

Findings in the Eye. Tuberculous diseases of the eye are rare (Weeks, 1926). The tuberculous allergic manifestation is more common than is infection by tubercle bacilli.

Phlyctenules of the conjunctiva and cornea are the commonest manifestations of tuberculous allergy, especially in the glandular type of tuberculosis. Phlyctenulosis was a common childhood disease in Alaska, and is still prevelant in (Fritz and Thygeson, 1954) underdeveloped countries. It is usually associated with enlargement of the tonsils and adenoids, swelling of the cervical lymphatic glands, eczema, and catarrh of various mucosa. In some countries it is still a principal cause of blindness. There are several clinical entities of phlyctenules, with such common symptoms as severe photophobia and blepharospasmus, itching, and often secondary bacterial infection, particularly staphylococcal.

PHLYCTENULAR CONJUNCTIVITIS.   The limbus is a site of phlyctenules. They are gray or pinkish white elevations vascularized on the periphery, which ulcerate easily. They are solitary nodular, often multiple, miliary elevations (Plate 11, Fig. 1), sometimes involving the entire limbal area. Ring ulcer may result. Ulceration of the phlyctenules is the basic feature differentiating them from other circumscribed lesions of the limbus, such as the limbal form of vernal conjunctivitis, rosacea, and pinguecula. The process usually heals without a trace but tends to recur.

PHLYCTENULAR KERATITIS.   The phlyctenules are situated predominantly in the exposed area of the cornea, either peripherally or centrally. They represent vascular or avascular circumscribed lesions having a tendency to necrotize, with resulting deep ulceration. Perforation may occur. In undernourished children the keratitis may become pustular and perforated (Plate 11, Fig. 3), due to secondary bacterial invasion, particularly staphylococcal. Leukoma adhaerens, anterior staphyloma, and blindness are the consequences. In less severe keratitis, single or multiple maculae remain and, if central, decrease vision.

Fascicular keratitis is manifested by a migrating phlyctenule pulling a vascular tail along the surface of the cornea. The movement can start at the limbus, moving toward the center, or it may cross the entire cornea in the form of a narrow, vascular ribbon (Plate 11, Fig. 2).

Phlyctenular (eczematous, scrofulous) pannus, unlike trachomatous pannus, may develop in any peripheral part of the cornea, mainly the lower, and in a late state of phlyctenules (Plate 11, Fig. 4).

Tubercle bacilli have not been demonstrated in any phlyctenular disease. In a scraping from the involved area, eosinophils may be present. Zalzman nodular degeneration occurs as a late consequence of chronic phlyctenular keratitis. The nodules are whitish and slowly progressive, resembling hyaline degeneration.

External eye infections caused by tubercle bacilli themselves are rare. They usually develop secondarily, either by continuity or by metastasis from other parts of the body. Occasionally, tuberculosis of the eye can be primary.

LUPUS VULGARIS. The process is the most common type of skin tuberculosis. The lid skin, conjunctiva, cornea, and lacrimal sac can be involved by continuation from adjacent tissue. Tuberculous ulcers of the lid margin resembling carcinoma, or nodules resembling chalazion, may occur.

CHRONIC DACRYOCYSTITIS. In young children, particularly girls, this is often a continuation of adjacent bone tuberculosis, or it can be primary.

TUBERCULOUS DACRYOADENITIS AND TUBERCULOSIS OF THE ORBITAL BONE. Both are usually of metastatic origin, are painless, with mild inflammatory reactions, and in the later stage, are characterized by fistula.

In all these processes, the finding of tubercle bacilli may often help establish the diagnosis.

KERATITIS DUE TO *M. TUBERCULOSIS*. Tuberculous infection of the cornea is mainly of metastatic origin. The resultant type of keratitis is typically deep nodular and may be abscesslike, often involving the upper external quadrant (Plate 10, Fig. 2) (as seen also in leprotic keratitis). The process is usually unilateral. As the cornea is a poor culture medium for the tubercle bacilli, the latter are very rarely found in tuberculous keratitis, and diagnosis is thus based mainly on the typical clinical picture. However, this type of keratitis could be an allergic manifestation. One also finds a diffuse interstitial keratitis, which is probably an anaphylactic phenomenon.

PRIMARY TUBERCULOSIS OF THE CONJUNCTIVA. This usually occurs in the palpebral conjunctiva. It is of exogenous origin, due to direct invasion by tubercle bacilli. A few clinical types are distinguished: ulcerative, hyperplastic, and mixed. The hyperplastic variety is subdivided into nodular and papillary types. The nodules appear as yellowish gray granules resembling those of trachoma. In the papillary type, the papillae may become pedunculated, and ulcers usually develop on the tops of the papillae (Plate 10, Fig. 1). A polypoidal type, or tuberculoma, has been described.

The common characteristics of the above types are the finding of tubercle bacilli in scrapings or histologic sections and an oculoglandular Parinaud's syndrome (swelling of the regional lymph glands).

The uveal tract and retina may be involved, usually in adults. Acute tuberculous panophthalmitis (Darrel) was caused by the tubercle bacillus in a patient without active tuberculosis. However, the history revealed pulmonary tuberculosis 40 years previously.

When tuberculosis of the inner eye is suspected, careful tuberculin testing must be used to avoid hypersensitivity reactions which can be dangerous for the eye.

Treatment. Combined treatment with streptomycin, para-aminosalicylic acid (PAS), and isonicotinic acid hydrazide (INH) greatly reduced mortality but does not prevent the infections. Most successful is combined treatment: INH with streptomycin and other antibiotics. Treatment is not always successful. This can be explained by the intracellular habitat of the bacilli, caseation, and a cavity with a fibrosed wall inhibiting drug penetration and action. In metastatic ocular tuberculosis, systemic treatment is required. This may also be indicated for primary ocular tuberculosis. The usual topical treatment for keratitis or iritis must be added. In allergic manifestations, the effect of cautious use of cortisone can be prompt.

Since resistance and hypersensitivity are decisive in tuberculous diseases, care of the general health may be even more important than the drug treatment. Host resistance can be reduced by many nonspecific factors, such as high doses of corticosteroids, immunosuppressive drugs, gastrectomy, and heavy smoking. Proper diet, good hygiene, fresh air, sufficient rest, and other factors are important in prevention and treatment. The incidence of disease is higher in an economically disadvantaged and crowded population area.

Mycobacterium leprae

The ancient, still dreaded disease, leprosy, is also called Hansen's disease, after Gerhard Hansen who, in 1874, reported his discovery of *M. leprae.*

Endemic areas of leprosy are found in most parts of the world (Richardson). There are approximately 2000 known cases of leprosy in the United States (Florida, Louisiana, Texas, Hawaii, and New York City). However, it is fairly common in tropical and subtropical regions.

Leprosy is a slowly progressive, chronic, granulomatous disease affecting skin, mucous membranes, peripheral nerves, and usually the lymph nodes. The portal of entry is probably the skin and nasal mucosa. The incubation period is of indefinite length, from two weeks to many years. Children are most sensitive to the infection but seldom develop symptoms of leprosy until adulthood. Since the mode of transmission is uncertain, segregation of infected persons in leprosaria is still practiced. As a prophylactic measure, it is recommended that children be segregated from their leprous parents.

Morphology.   The bacilli are pleomorphic and acid-fast, resembling tubercle bacilli. Morphologically, they resemble diphtheroids, varying in size and in shape from long, straight, or curved to irregular coccoid or granular forms (Plate 12, Fig. 4). They decolorize more readily (by Ziehl-Neelsen) than do tubercle bacilli, and are arranged in clumps, bundles, palisades, or globular masses. The organisms are regularly found in scrapings, especially in the nodular form of leprosy. They grow best intracellularly in endothelial and mononuclear cells. The role of the bacillus as sole etiologic agent is not completely established. The bacilli have never been cultivated, but they have undergone limited multiplication when inoculated into the footpads of mice (Shepard).

Serologic tests are of no value.

Pathology.   Leprosy is characterized by the production of leproma (granuloma), diffuse infiltration, or both. Pathologic examination reveals connective tissue cells, many plasma cells, and a conglomerate of lepra cells (large, poorly defined masses) loaded with bacilli (in the nodular form). The cells probably are degenerated giant cells.

The pathology of ocular leprosy has been described by Allen and Byers.

Clinical Features.   Clinical manifestations of leprosy vary greatly. The clinical symptoms may differ even in the same geographic area, or they can be common in different clinical forms of leprosy. Therefore, several clinical or pathologic divisions have been proposed. In practice, two divisions are most acceptable: (1) the nodular lepromatous form and (2) the neural anesthetic tuberculoid form (also called maculoanesthetic). Both forms can be present in the same patient. In the nodular type, lesions appear on the exposed skin surfaces, ie, hands and face, especially on the nose (Plate 12, Fig. 2), forehead, and lips (causing the characteristic lionlike faces). This is a contagious form, and bacilli are constantly found.

The neural (maculoanesthetic) form is characterized by diffuse infiltration of peripheral nerves (chronic interstitial neuritis), with consequent loss of sensation. Therefore the hands and feet are easily damaged, often with resultant grotesque deformation. A clawlike appearance of the hands (Plate 12, Fig. 6) may develop because of nerve and muscle atrophy. The cell response is the same as in the nodular form, except that bacilli are very few and are difficult to find.

Findings in the Eye.   Leprosy may involve any or all of the ocular structures. The incidence of ocular involvement may be 75 to 90 percent (Elliot; Harley; Kennedy).

Corneal involvement is common (Allen and Byers) and is the main cause of blindness in lepers. Three main clinical forms of leprotic keratitis are distinguished: (1) leprotic superficial punctate keratitis, (2) leprotic pannus in the upper half, similar to trachomatous (or in the outer quadrant of the cornea), and (3) interstitial keratitis. These forms may represent one process in its different stages. The common characteristics of the three are corneal anesthesia, thickening of the nerves in the stroma, scattered, chalky, minute grains (Plate 12, Fig. 1), the presence of the organisms, and no tendency to ulceration. Sometimes, a very destructive process in the form of a tumorlike leproma invades and destroys the entire cornea. Corneal leproma (Plate 12, Fig. 5) shows a yellowish mass with deep vascularization. The process is indolent and symptomless, resembling an old scar. The nodules may show central necrosis, which sometimes results in the formation of ulcer, perforation, and staphyloma.

The lids are frequently affected. The nodular type of leprosy may typically involve the skin of the upper lids but usually spares the lower lids and lid margins. However, in the area adjacent to the nodules, the lashes fall out.

The conjunctiva is rarely affected. In nodular leprosy, miliary, yellowish, or white nodules develop, usually at the upper outer quadrant of the limbus, more rarely in the bulbar conjunctiva. The nodules may ulcerate, and the process often spreads into the cornea and the sclera.

Paralysis of the orbicularis muscle may occur in neural maculoanesthetic leprosy. Ulcerative keratitis, papillary conjunctivitis, and fleshy pterygium may result secondary to the lagophthalmos.

Leprosy predominantly involves the anterior segment of the eye. However, the posterior segment may be affected, and, according to Pendergast, fundus changes took place in 42 out of 241 patients. The case illustrated (Plate 12, Fig. 3) showed a group of discrete lesions in the periphery of the fundus, resembling the picture reported by Trantas. Elliot reported six cases of retinal pearls visible through the ophthalmoscope. These have been described as superficial nodules in the retina. Granulomatous uveitis, with tissue necrosis and enormous numbers of bacilli, has been recorded.

Treatment.   No specific treatment is known. It is extremely important to pay attention to the general health. Antituberculosis treatment may have some effect, and the use of streptomycin or the sulfones Promin and Diasone has been reported as helpful. A long period of treatment, from two to nine years, is required.

Other Mycobacteria (Atypical)

As a result of new drug treatment of tuberculosis there has been an increase in the number of atypical mycobacteria, which can produce infections that can be confused with tuberculosis. Fifty percent of people in the southeastern part of the United States have been infected by these atypical, so-called anonymous, mycobacteria. The most common is lymphadenitis or skin granuloma in children, which is not contagious. Their taxonomic and medical significance is not fully established. Description of their grouping (Runyon) can be found in

Jawetz E, Melnick JL, Adelberg EA: *The Review of Medical Microbiology*, 2nd edition, 1974.

Diagnosis is based on their resistance to antituberculosis treatment, particularly streptomycin, on histologic examination of the lesions, and on bacteriologic culture.

This group of acid-fast mycobacteria includes saprophytes in a free environment, the organisms causing disease in domestic animals (cattle), and *Mycobacterium marinum*, a cause of swimming pool granuloma in man. Others are found in man's sebaceous exudate. Most of these can grow on simple media even at 22C, producing significant pigment and being resistant to antituberculosis treatment.

Findings in the Eye. Several cases of infection due to anonymous mycobacteria have been reported in ophthalmic literature: stromal keratitis resembling keratomycosis (Lauring et al), two cases of acute corneal ulcers, one following injury by a foreign body, the second a penetrating keratoplasty (Zimmerman et al). Avian tuberculosis endophthalmitis of Wasserman can be considered as atypical mycobacterial infection. It is highly resistant to chemical treatment.

GRAM–NEGATIVE GROUP

NEISSERIACEAE

The members of this family are gram-negative cocci, typically intracellular and arranged in pairs. Except in the case of the gonococcus, they are normal inhabitants of the nasopharynx in man, healthy or ill. The genera discussed here are *Neisseria, Branhamella (N. catarrhaeis), Moraxella,* and *Acinetobacter* (Mimeae).

Neisseria gonorrhoeae

The gonococcus was first described by Neisser in 1879, when he isolated the organism from purulent urethritis and vaginitis. Gonorrhea is the most prevalent of the venereal diseases. The sensitivity of the gonococcus to sulfonamides and penicillin has greatly decreased the incidence of acute infection. However, resistant strains are no longer rare. More important is the fact that the disease may become chronic in persons who seem to have been cured and in whom laboratory tests reveal no organisms. The incidence of asymptomatic gonorrhea in females is very high.

Extragenital gonococcal infection may occur: cystitis, stomatitis, and more often, conjunctivitis in the newborn (ophthalmia neonatorum).

The infection may invade the blood, and septicemia, arthritis, and endocarditis are among the sequelae.

Morphology. Smears reveal N. *gonorrhoeae* to be mainly a typical kidney-shaped diplococcus. Isolated cocci and those from cultures are round, resembling staphylococci. While N. *gonorrhoeae* may be found extracellularly, usually in a chronic process, intracellular occurrence within leukocytes is more characteristic and is important for diagnosis (Plate 13, Fig. 3A). The organism stains readily with methylene blue alone. Difficulties arise with the gram stain because gonococci are not always readily decolorized, or the involution forms found in culture are often swollen and take the stain poorly (Plate 13, Fig. 3B). The organisms retaining stain may be mistaken for staphylococci. *Acinetobacter* (Mimeae) also appears on smear as gram-negative intracellular diplococci, but it appears typically in chronic conditions. To obtain a good stain, one must prepare as thin and uniform a film as possible. This will allow a microscopic diagnosis of the smear secretion.

Immunofluorescent staining of smears is more efficient, particularly in asymptomatic cases of gonorrhea.

Culture. The gonococci require enriched media. While many different media are used, growth may be obtained with the simplest of them, such as chocolate or blood agar, particularly in an atmosphere containing 10 percent carbon dioxide. The carbon dioxide atmosphere can be produced within a candle jar. Since the gonococci require moisture, a piece of moist blotting paper should be placed on the bottom of the jar along with the inoculated plate. Thayer-Martin medium is used for improving the growth and inhibiting other bacteria in mixed culture. The gonococci are easily autolyzed and die rapidly, hence incubation should not be longer than 48 hours. They grow best at a slightly lower than normal incubation temperature, 35 to 36 C. The material should be swabbed into a broth and brought to the laboratory immediately, then inoculated, as gonococci die rapidly at room temperature.

On chocolate agar, colonies are unpigmented, glistening, large, mucoid, and semitranslucent. They have irregular edges, do not produce hemolysis, and are odorless.

Members of the *Neisseria* genus produce oxidase and autolytic enzymes. Therefore, the oxidase test is used to identify colonies of the *Neisseria* genus and to distinguish them in mixed, overcrowded plates. For the test, the dye solution (1 percent of dimethyl or tetramethyl para-phenylenediamine) must be dropped on the suspicious area. The oxidase-positive colonies turn from pink to red to black. When the color is black, the organism is dead (Plate 14, Fig. 5). Some of the gram-negative bacilli show a positive oxidase test, but their color is gray instead of black.

For differential diagnosis of the species, the fermentation test is necessary. The gonococcus ferments glucose but does not ferment maltose or sucrose (Plate 13, Fig. 6).

Antigenic Structure.   It is difficult to establish definite serologic types, since the majority of strains are antigenically related. There are, however, two main antigenic types: type I, usually involved in an acute process, and type II, in chronic processes. Between these two there are a number of intermediate types containing one or more common antigens.

Gonococcal polysaccharides and nucleoproteins are not specific and are similar to those of the meningococcus. Permanent immunity does not develop.

Pathogenicity and Virulence.   The gonococcus is very restricted as to its human portal of entry. It attacks mainly the mucous membranes of the genitourinary tract and the conjunctiva. The disease process is acutely purulent and usually local. Blood invasion occurs rarely, and arthritis (very painful), endocarditis with skin hemorrhagic lesions, or other conditions may develop, all probably of toxic origin.

The gonococcus produces an endotoxin that can be extracted from the organisms. The endotoxin may be liberated from the culture by autolysis of the bacteria.

The resistance of the gonococcus is very low. It is easily destroyed by drying and by heat, even as low as 30 C, within five minutes.

Findings in the Eye.   Recently there has been a striking increase in the number of acute cases of gonococcal conjunctivitis, particularly in a new age group—teen-agers. This conjunctivitis is often associated with a high incidence of gonorrhea. The gonococcus may cause a violent acute purulent conjunctivitis, which may be complicated by ulceration of the cornea, with resultant scarring and blindness. Two main age types are clinically distinguished: gonococcal conjunctivitis of the newborn (ophthalmia neonatorum) and gonococcal conjunctivitis of the adult.

GONOCOCCAL CONJUNCTIVITIS IN THE NEWBORN (OPHTHALMIA NEONATORUM). While this condition is not common where the law requires prophylaxis, it may still develop (Baraff). It results from gonorrheal urethritis of the mother. The infant's eyes are infected during the passage through the birth canal. Extremely rarely does ocular infection occur in utero. The incubation period of ophthalmia neonatorum is one to three days, and involvement is usually bilateral. At onset there is a sanious discharge, which then becomes purulent (Plate 13, Fig. 2) and so copious that it may flow down the cheek. Sometimes pseudomembranes may develop. The markedly swollen lids are difficult to open, and pus accumulates in the conjunctival sac. Glasses should be worn while opening the child's lids, or pus may spray into the observer's eyes and cause a severe ocular infection. In spite of the copious purulent discharge, the conjunctival tissue may at first be only slightly involved.

Later, it becomes very red and rough. On this basis, gonococcal conjunctivitis is differentiated from the other bacterial conjunctivitides in the newborn. For example, in staphylococcal infections, the conjunctiva is only slightly involved.

Gonococcal ophthalmia, particularly in severe or untreated cases, is commonly complicated by a severe purulent type of keratitis. It is associated with the period of discharge and marked edema of the lids. The pressure by the swollen lids decreases the blood supply, and toxic pus macerates the corneal epithelium, thus creating a portal of entry. The keratitis begins as a yellowish infiltrate, which progresses and ulcerates very rapidly, with resulting perforation and panophthalmitis.

The disease is highly contagious, and isolation of the child is mandatory.

In children's hospital wards, schools, or orphanages, epidemics of vulvovaginitis or infantile purulent conjunctivitis may occur. The conjunctivitis can be caused by staphylococci, streptococci, or other bacteria, but the gonococcus is the prime offender. It usually occurs in girls aged 2 to 10, transmitted by direct sexual contact or deviation. In our laboratory, the gonococcus was isolated from a sporadic case of infantile purulent conjunctivitis in a 5-year-old girl (Plate 13, Fig. 1). Nonvenereal transmission of gonococcal infection of children 6 to 12 years old was found in Alaska (Shore and Winkelstein). The contact was not established. Laboratory examination is essential for differential diagnosis.

GONOCOCCAL CONJUNCTIVITIS IN THE ADULT. This condition is usually unilateral and results from self-transmission of the organism from the urethral tract (Plate 13, Fig. 4). Therefore, it occurs mainly in males, and the right eye is most frequently involved. The clinical picture, while similar to ophthalmia neonatorum, has certain differences: the purulent discharge is not as copious, and the conjunctival tissue tends to be more involved and becomes more papillary and rougher than in children. The most important characteristic is that the cornea is almost constantly involved in untreated cases. A marginal ulcer is the most common type and may take the form of a ring, resulting in perforation. Until the antibiotic era, many eyes were lost. As in children, the possible consequences are perforation of the cornea, endophthalmitis, and panophthalmitis. Even now, the prognosis in adults must be guarded.

Iritis, iridocyclitis with hypopyon (without involvement of the cornea), or lid abscess may develop.

Prophylaxis. The classical prophylaxis by Credé, proposed in 1880, consisted of instillation of one drop of 1 percent silver nitrate solution into each eye of the newborn. Its requirement by law in most parts of the world brought a great advance in the prevention of gonococcal conjunctivitis. The method has recently been reevaluated because of irritation by the silver nitrate, and prophylaxis by antibiotics has been advocated (Lewis, 1946). However, a new problem arose: sensitivity of the host to antibiotics, especially penicillin. As a result some go as far as to omit any prophylaxis, since antibiotic action is specific for gonococcal infection, which may be easily treated. However, an increase of gonococcal conjunctivitis in the newborn has been reported. Therefore, prophylaxis still is the accepted procedure.

If silver nitrate is used, the lid margin first must be thoroughly cleansed with dry cotton, then the silver nitrate instilled. It is important that this be in contact with the entire conjunctiva. Silver nitrate may prevent *Herpes virus simplex* Type 1 infection in the newborn.

In adults' conjunctivitis, the unaffected eye should be protected by Buller's or some other shield.

Diagnosis. The typical clinical picture and study of a properly prepared smear may be satisfactory for diagnosis. The organisms are more easily seen in the beginning period of purulent discharge. For early diagnosis of gonoccal conjunctivitis, particularly in adults, scraping is preferable to smear. It shows gonococci on the epithelial cells prior to finding them in the secretion (Plate 13, Fig. 5). A culture is necessary in a case of negative smear and in order to confirm the diagnosis. Gonococci may remain in the conjunctiva after the clinical symptoms disappear.

Treatment. Since the accumulation of pus aids corneal involvement by maceration of the epithelium, it is highly recommended that in the period of copious purulent discharge the eyes should be washed constantly. Saline or other solutions can be used. Strains resistant to penicillin and the sulfonamides, which were so effective in the past, have now developed. However, penicillin is still the drug of choice, with sulfonamides for local use. Ampicillin appears to be highly effective in cases of penicillin resistance (Spaeth). Oral tetracycline, erythromycin, and neomycin have all been used successfully, though resistance to these antibiotics can also develop.

Neisseria meningitidis

The meningococcus is of great importance in medicine, as it causes epidemics of cerebrospinal meningitis, which can often be fatal. Man is the only known natural host of pathogenic meningococci. These intracellular diplococci have a morphology similar to that of the gonococcus (Plate 14, Fig. 2). Cultural requirements and characteristics are also similar (Plate 14, Fig. 3) except that the meningococcus ferments glucose and maltose but not sucrose (Plate 14, Fig. 4).

The meningococci have been separated into four major groups, A, B, C, and D, corresponding to the old classification of types I, II, III, and IV. Group D is rarely found in the United States. Groups A and C have capsules that react with specific antisera and result in Quellung similar to that found in the pneumococcus. There are additional groups known as X, Y, and Z. Each type may be identified through agglutination tests with specific sera, valuable only in time of epidemic. Infants have passive immunity by transference of IgG antibody from the mother.

Pathogenicity and Virulence. The nucleoproteins of *N. meningitidis* are regarded as endotoxins, but they are not specific. Toxicity is probably caused by some constituents of the nucleoproteins. No immunity develops.

Pathology. The meningococcus is a specific cause of purulent epidemic cerebrospinal meningitis, especially in children. Epidemics have a tendency to cyclic occurrence at about 8 to 12 year intervals. The most severe cases occur in adults, especially soldiers. A severe outbreak in the United States was recorded at the beginning of World War II (1940–43).

If the organisms reach the bloodstream, meningococcemia develops, which is usually characterized by purpuric spots, due to thrombosis of the capillaries. Meningococci may be cultured from these spots, especially in an early stage. Meningococcemia may become chronic.

The source of infection is usually a healthy carrier or a person who has recovered from the disease. The nasopharynx is the major portal and harbor of infection. In persons who have been exposed to the infection, the nasopharynx must be examined and treated during an epidemic.

Findings in the Eye. Meningococcal ocular infections are discussed increasingly in the literature. In 1944 and 1946, a considerable number of cases were reported (Mangiaracine and Pollen; Odegaard; Reid and Bronstein; Theodore and Kost, 1944). Acute conjunctivitis is the most common manifestation. This is purulent, sometimes resembling gonococcal conjunctivitis, and occasionally occurs in the newborn. The conjunctivitis may be complicated by various types of keratitis, among which are mild ulceration and multiple stromal infiltration. In a case reported by Allen, the latter showed peripheral diffuse circular bands. More rarely, endophthalmitis may develop. It has been recorded that bilateral meningococcal endophthalmitis developed in 7-year-old girls who had meningococcemia (Jensen and Naidoff). Free meningococci have been reported in a case of keratomalacia. In our laboratory, meningococci were isolated from pus of opened meibomitis. Another patient, a boy of 12, developed mild purulent meningococcal conjunctivitis and a few stromal infiltrates of the cornea (Plate 14, Fig. 1). The laboratory investigation of material from the inflamed meibomian gland seemed reasonable. It is probable that the glands can harbor meningococci.

The ocular condition may occur independently or as a complication of the meningitis (Kahaner and Lanou). Papillitis is most frequently found, and among the other complications, retinitis, subconjunctival hemorrhages, and endophthalmitis may occur. On the other hand, infection from the eye can invade the blood, causing meningococcemia and meningitis.

It must be stressed that meningococcal ocular infection is much more frequent than is realized (Crabb et al). Meningococci can also be found in normal flora, being a potential source of infection. Therefore, complete study of the culture and serologic differentiation of the *Neisseria* species is important.

Treatment.   The meningococcus is becoming resistant to the sulfa drugs with which meningococcal infection was treated almost universally. Today a high percentage of organisms isolated in meningitis are sulfa-resistant. Penicillin in high doses is usually effective treatment, although some resistant strains have developed. Even in those cases in which conjunctivitis is the only manifestation of meningococcal infection, local therapy plus intensive systemic treatment by sulfadiazine or penicillin should be employed to prevent meningitis. During epidemics, it is advisable to investigate the normal flora of the conjunctiva of persons exposed, and if meningococci are found, the introduction of sulfonamides, especially of sulfadiazine ointment, may be useful for prophylaxis.

Branhamella catarrhalis

Branhamella catarrhalis (previously named *Neisseria catarrhalis*) is a constant inhabitant of the respiratory tract. It is generally considered saprophytic, but it can at times be weakly pathogenic. *B. catarrhalis* may be confused with *N. meningitidis*, since both are inhabitants of the pharynx, and differential diagnosis is of great importance.

Morphologically in the smear secretion it is indistinguishable from gonococci and meningococci. It is coffee-bean-shaped and intracellular (Plate 15, Fig. 1). Nonetheless, these cocci may be larger than the neisseria and may stain more intensely.

Cultural differentiation is most significant. *B. catarrhalis*, unlike the neisseria, grows abundantly and freely on ordinary media (Plate 15, Fig. 5). On plain agar the colonies are round, gray, and glistening, but after 24 hours of incubation, they become opaque and slightly brown in the center. Their tendency to autoagglutinate makes it practically impossible to achieve a uniform suspension.

Biochemically, *B. catarrhalis* does not produce acid or gas from any of the sugars. Fermentation tests with maltose, glucose, and sucrose are negative. *B. catarrhalis* is more resistant to physical agents than are gonococci and meningococci.

Findings in the Eye. Although principally nonpathogenic, *B. catarrhalis* may become a pathogen in certain eye conditions. It is occasionally found in mild and even severe cases of conjunctivitis and in postoperative conjunctivitis. The organism is found most frequently in cases of inflammation of the meibomian glands.

An extremely rare case of endophthalmitis due to *B. catarrhalis* has been reported (Givner).

Fermentation Tests

For differentiation of *N. gonorrhoeae*, *N. meningitidis*, and *B. catarrhalis*, fermentation tests are most important:

	MALTOSE	GLUCOSE	SUCROSE
Neisseria gonorrhoeae	−	+	−
Neisseria meningitidis	+	+	−
Branhamella catarrhalis	−	−	−

B. catarrhalis is further distinguished by the fact that it grows on ordinary media.

Moraxella lacunata

This organism was discovered by Morax in 1896 and independently by Axenfeld in 1897. It, therefore, became known as the Morax-Axenfeld diplobacillus. In 1939 the genus *Moraxella* was established by Lwoff. The species of interest here are *Moraxella lacunata*, *Moraxella* subsp. *liquefaciens* (originally called the diplobacillus of Petit), *Moraxella nonliquefaciens*, and *Moraxella bovis*. Although van Bijsterveld (1973) placed them in no family, the 8th edition of *Bergey's Manual* includes them in the Neisseriaceae.

M. lacunata is responsible only for ocular diseases, and therefore general bacteriologists have given it little attention. It was originally considered a principal cause of chronic angular blepharoconjunctivitis.

Morphology. *M. lacunata* is the largest gram-negative bacillus causing ocular diseases. The variation in stain is typical. The organism often retains the gram-positive stain, and in the same slide, both gram-positive and gram-negative bacilli can be seen. The long diplobacilli usually stain pale pink, whereas the short, stout coccobacilli may be gram-positive. In secretion the bacilli are short but stout, with intensively staining rectangular or round ends (polar stain). While usually arranged in pairs, hence diplobacilli, the organisms may at times appear in short chains, and capsules may be present (Plate 16, Fig. 3B). The secretion is characteristically mucoid, with fibrin threads, and it is not purulent. Numerous organisms are usually found, either free or within epithelial cells, even in the mild, almost asymptomatic process. *M. lacunata* may proliferate on the surface of desquamated epithelium. This organism has a typical morphology in secretion, and thus diagnosis is possible from a study of the smear alone. The morphology changes quickly in culture (Plate 16, Figs. 3A, 5). Only during the first day can one find typical diplobacillary or streptobacillary forms. Later, one may find forms varying from very long, thin filaments resembling fungi to short coccobacilli or ovoid bodies. The variations in this respect are so marked that in our laboratory, we have demonstrated a linkage to the micrococcus described by Mitsui, Hinokuma, and Tanaka (Horwich and Fedukowicz). Sometimes the cells of *M. lacunata* become club-shaped, thus resembling corynebacteria.

The organisms are nonmotile, nonsporeforming aerobes.

Culture. *M. lacunata* requires enriched media and prefers an alkaline environment. Generally it grows on any medium containing animal serum. Löffler's medium is certainly the most practical for the ophthalmologist. Pits are formed on this medium, demonstrating the degree of liquefaction, an important characteristic for identification (Plate 16, Fig. 4). While no actual colonies are visible on the medium, the surface is covered by circumscribed pits of liquefaction, hence the term *lacunata*. On blood agar, the colonies develop slowly. They are grayish, semitransparent, mucoid, usually nonhemolytic, and odorless. Others are pinpoint, translucent, dewdrop in appearance, and easy to overlook. They are more typical for *M. lacunata* subsp. *liquefaciens*. A carbon dioxide, wet atmosphere improves growth. There is no growth of *M. lacunata* on chocolate agar, and there is no fermentation of sugars. *M. lacunata* grows in symbiosis with *C. xerosis*, an organism that does not produce any acid. It usually does not grow well in the presence of the acid-producing *S. aureus*. In our experience, *S. aureus* is rarely found in direct smear when *M. lacunata* is present.

Resistance. According to the literature, these diplobacilli usually die after about 10 days of subcultivation. In our laboratory, we have been able to keep cultures alive for almost three weeks by transferring them every other day. Without transference they die quickly. *M. lacunata* can be killed in one to five minutes by moist heat at 58 C.

Pathogenicity.   As far as is known, *M. lacunata* causes the typical clinical picture of angular blepharoconjunctivitis or hypopyon keratitis. It is suggested that these diplobacilli produce the enzyme, protease, which can be inhibited by tears (believed to contain antiprotease). Hence, it is possible that bacilli try to escape to the angulus from the conjunctiva, which is bathed in tears. Angular blepharoconjunctivitis then develops. However, no correlation between the amount or type of protease and the location of the maceration was found by van Bijsterveld (1971).

White mice may die within 24 hours after intraperitoneal injection of a suspension of *M. lacunata* (Oeding). However, animal passage has not been successful. We have observed that intracorneal inoculation of strains isolated from hypopyon keratitis produces a deep hypopyon keratitis in rabbits (Fedukowicz, Alterman, and Newman).

Findings in the Eye.   Chronic angular blepharoconjunctivitis is an almost pathognomonic indication for *M. lacunata* infection (Axenfeld). While rare in most of the United States, the disease is not uncommon in Arizona and New Mexico. Epidemics have occurred, but they have not been severe. In general the condition is endemic, particularly in institutions (personal observations in institutions for the retarded). The disease affects predominantly adults, during hot dusty seasons or in hot climates, although cases have been reported in the newborn. *Moraxella* organisms were found frequently in the nasal swabs of alcoholics. The nose seems to be the natural habitat of *Moraxella* (van Bijsterveld, 1972).

Blepharoconjunctivitis is a chronic process which may last for years. It is characterized by redness, particularly of the outer anguli (Plate 16, Fig. 1). Numerous diplobacilli can be isolated from this site, even in very mild conditions. These mild cases may easily be overlooked and, if untreated, may cause postoperative infections.

Moraxella bacilli very rarely causes a severe acute conjunctivitis.

We observed an unusual follicular conjunctivitis, which runs an acute or chronic course, in epidemic proportions among schoolgirls who applied heavy mascara and who shared the mascara. Scrapings showed typical diplobacilli in nearly all cases. In the majority, the diagnosis was confirmed by positive culture. *Chlamydia* (TRIC agents) and allergy were ruled out by the absence of pannus and cytologic study of the scrapings. The long-lasting constant mechanical irritation by the mascara could contribute to the follicular response.

The cornea may show a marginal type of ulceration similar to any other ulcer associated with bacterial conjunctivitis.

Severe stormy keratitis, in our observations, contradicts the dominant conception of ophthalmologists that *Moraxella* keratitis is mild and painless. We had a unique opportunity to observe 85 different varieties of keratitis in 85 cases of *Moraxella* infection, as reported in 1970 (Fedukowicz et al).

A central hypopyon keratitis, typically in abscess form, may occur primarily (without preceding blepharoconjunctivitis), particularly in elderly male alcoholics and debilitated persons (Plate 16, Fig. 2). A history of preceding ocular trauma was commonly elicited. Hypopyon keratitis due to *Moraxella diplobacillus* is the predominant type found at Bellevue Hospital, in contrast to the high incidence of pneumococcal keratitis reported elsewhere (Fedukowicz and Horwich). The process spreads deeply, possibly to avoid contact with tears, and often painlessly, with development of an intracorneal abscess. Sometimes two zones of infiltration are seen: a central one separated by a clear area from a peripheral one. A posterior abscess may occur. Some appear to be similar to a neuroparalytic ulcer, with a little exudation, absence of corneal sensitivity, and presence of numerous typical *Moraxella diplobacillus* in scrapings.

At onset, the surface of the cornea over the abscess may appear intact. Later, necrosis and ulceration develop. Scraping the cornea is of value only after the cornea breaks down. First the necrotic mass is cleaned away, then the ulcer base must be scraped, since it is here that the bacilli reside (not in the margin, as in the case of pneumococcal ulcer). Perforation of the cornea or secondary glaucoma may often result.

Treatment. Zinc salts appear to have an almost specific action upon *Moraxella* infections. In cases of blepharoconjunctivitis, a 0.25 percent to 0.5 percent solution of zinc sulfate, three times a day, can be recommended. To treat keratitis in the preantibiotic era, zinc sulfate in high concentrations was used, but with extreme caution and only if the cornea was not too thinned by the process. Cauterization with 5 or 10 percent solution of zinc sulfate can be effective in the early stages of keratitis, particularly if antibiotics are not effective or are not available. In this technique, the following steps should be followed: The eye must be thoroughly anesthetized topically, since cauterization is a painful procedure. For cauterization, a thin applicator is necessary; a wooden toothpick will suffice. The applicator must be only dampened, and any excess of the solution must be avoided. The cautery is applied only to the involved site, with care not to touch normal cornea. The cauterized tissue turns white, and this is an indication to stop the procedure immediately. A second treatment may be given in a day or two. Meanwhile, drops of 0.5 or 0.25 percent zinc sulfate solution should be used three times a day. The physician should be aware that severe pain usually follows, in which case systemic pain medication is indicated.

Sulfonamides, streptomycin, tetracyclines, or neomycin are used depending upon the results of antibiotic sensitivity tests. Surgical procedures, including Saemisch's section, Sondermann's trephination, and delimiting keratotomy, have been used. These procedures may reduce the tension and bring additional antibodies from the secondary aqueous.

In our department, keratoplasty (lamellar or, in a deep process, perforating) has been successful in saving the eye.

Enzymatic debridement can be effective.

Supportive measures, such as a good diet with vitamin B supplement, should be given, especially when the patient is alcoholic or otherwise debilitated.

Moraxella lacunata subsp. liquefaciens

In 1899, Petit isolated an organism from three cases of purulent keratitis. On the basis of clinical and laboratory evidence, he considered this to be a distinct entity, although it had some similarity to *M. lacunata.*

From a clinical point of view, he believed *M. lacunata* to be of low infectivity, able to cause only a mild process, such as angular blepharoconjunctivitis. When the diplobacillus had sufficiently high virulence to cause a severe hypopyon keratitis, he called it the "diplobacillus of Petit" (now *Moraxella lacunata* subsp. *liquefaciens).*

While Petit found these two diplobacilli to be indistinguishable morphologically (Plate 17, Fig. 2), he felt that their cultural characteristics were different. He declared that the Petit diplobacillus, unlike the Morax-Axenfeld diplobacillus, could grow on ordinary media (Plate 17, Fig. 4) and had the ability to liquefy Löffler's serum more effectively (Plate 17, Fig. 3).

His views greatly affected our concept of diplobacillary keratitis. The name Petit was linked with virtually every case of diplobacillary keratitis (Plate 17, Fig. 1). However, many cases of central hypopyon keratitis have been reported as being due to *M. lacunata,* and therefore much confusion has arisen. Later studies (van Bijsterveld, 1973) reveal that there is no serologic and only slight cultural difference between the organisms isolated from both clinical entities; hence, the name *M. lacunata* subsp. *liquefaciens.* Various investigators have grown both organisms on ordinary media.

In our observations, *M. lacunata* and *M. lacunata* subsp. *liquefaciens* were found equally often in hypopyon keratitis, conjunctivitis, and blepharoconjunctivitis.

Acinetobacter (Mimeae)

In 1942 de Bord described a group of organisms resembling *Neisseria* in some morphologic, enzymatic, and clinical aspects. Both are gram-negative diplococci and characteristically intracellular (Plate 15, Fig. 2). Therefore the name Mimeae was applied (it mimics *Neisseria*). It was found later that it mimics *Moraxella* as well as *Neisseria*. In the study of their relationships Henriksen made a great contribution, as did King, by adding more data about their biologic and serologic characteristics. As a result, a Mima-Moraxella group was created, with multiple common characteristics. In the 8th edition of *Bergey's Manual*, Mimeae are classified as the genus, *Acinetobacter*, with the single species, *Acinetobacter calcoaceticus*.

Laboratory Differential Diagnosis. The exact differentiation among *Acinetobacter*, *Moraxella*, and *Neisseria* is complicated, and a number of tests are required. For practical purposes, *Acinetobacter* can be separated out by the oxidase test: *Neisseria* and *Moraxella* are oxidase-positive, *Acinetobacter* is oxidase-negative. Another test is the morphologic differentiation in direct smear. *Moraxella* is a bacillus, *Neisseria* is a coccus, and *Acinetobacter* shows in culture very short rods and coccal forms (Plate 15, Fig. 3). The absence of a bacillary form in *Neisseria* is an important diferential characteristic. Additionally, *Acinetobacter* and *Moraxella* do not typically ferment sugars as does *Neisseria*, and *Acinetobacter* and *Neisseria* do not liquefy serum as does *Moraxella*.

The diagnosis of *Acinetobacter* infection should not be neglected when gonococcal infection is suspected, and it should be kept in mind that it has been confused with the gonococcus much more often than is realized (Plate 15, Fig. 2).

The cultural characteristics of *Acinetobacter* are not always distinctive. Growth can sometimes be abundant, and colonies with a dew-drop appearance similar to some *Moraxella* colonies, can be found.

Pathology and Pathogenesis. *Acinetobacter* is mostly saprophytic or mildly pathogenic and is found in normal flora, sputum, urine, and many mucous membranes. They become pathogenic in burns or in immunologic deficiency, and serious diseases, such as meningitis, endocarditis, and sepsis, are reported increasingly. *Acinetobacter* are weakly antigenic, and their serologic study has been most intensive. Ten or more serologic types are known.

Findings in the Eye. The organism that formed the basis of the Mimeae classification by de Bord was obtained from a prepuberty vagina, purulent conjunctivitis, and conjunctivitis neonatorum. Among our 85 cases of keratitis mentioned previously, *Acinetobacter* was isolated in 2 cases. *Moraxella nonliquefaciens* was found in 13 cases. Recently corneal perforation due to *Acinetobacter* in an 11-year-old girl was reported (Wand et al). This was associated with hyperacute conjunctivitis. Corneal marginal ulcer due to *Bacterium anitratum*, reclassified as *Acinetobacter* in the 8th edition of *Bergey's Manual*, has been recorded (Presley and Hale). In our laboratory *Acinetobacter* was isolated in 7 cases of follicular conjunctivitis (Plate 15, Fig. 4), and in 4 cases of ophthalmia neonatorum.

Treatment. *Acinetobacter* is sensitive to most antibiotics, such as tetracycline, kanamycin, and gentamycin, but it can develop resistance. It is characteristically resistant to penicillin, a helpful point for differential purposes.

THE *HAEMOPHILUS* GENUS

Haemophilus influenzae is the most important pathogen of this genus. It was described as the cause of influenza by Pfeiffer in 1893. Since that time many other members of the genus have been described, many of which are nonpathogenic. Among those pathogenic for man are *Haemophilus influenzae*, *Haemophilus ducreyi*, and *Haemophilus aegyptius* (the Koch-Weeks bacillus). *H. aegyptius*, strictly an ocular pathogen, is recognized by ophthalmologists as a species of the hemophilic group. It is very closely related to *H. influenzae*.

Haemophilus aegyptius

This bacillus was first described by Koch when, in 1884, he found it as a secondary invader in trachoma in Egypt.

Independently, Weeks in 1886 described the same bacillus as the cause of epidemic acute conjunctivitis in New York (Feldman). Since that time this type of conjunctivitis has been recognized along the coastlines of the United States and throughout Europe and Africa. It is very rare in Central America.

The Koch-Weeks bacillus is very common in Egypt, hence the name *H. aegyptius*. However, the name Koch-Weeks bacillus, is more familiar in ophthalmology. *H. aegyptius* frequently causes an infection superimposed on trachoma, and the entire process then resembles gonoblennorrhea.

Minton described epidemics of infective conjunctivitis in Iraq, Palestine, and Egypt. The epidemics usually occurred yearly (from May to August) among children. Ulceration of the cornea frequently complicated the conjunctivitis.

Morphology. Though typical in smear secretion, the organism is not easily found. The bacillus is minute, usually coccobacillary or a slender gram-negative rod. The bacilli take a very pale stain from safranin (counterstain by the gram method), and carbolfuchsin gives a better result. There is no characteristic arrangement, and the organisms may appear singly, in pairs, in short chains, or as tangled masses. In smear secretion the bacilli are found free or intracellularly within the leukocytes and epithelial cells. Because of their small size, they are adapted to an intracellular habitat. This can be well demonstrated in scrapings (Plate 18, Fig. 3B).

The morphology varies when the organism is cultured. The same strain can be so pleomorphic that it is difficult to recognize as the same organism. Wavy, curved, and very long filamentous forms develop in the culture (Plate 18, Fig. 3A). In young cultures on rich media, smooth (S) forms are encapsulated, but capsules are rarely found in an older culture.

A culture is necessary for diagnosis.

Culture. Both *H. influenzae* and *H. aegyptius* require both the X and V growth factors, which serve as a basis for the differentiation of *Haemophilus* strains, particularly *Haemophilus parainfluenzae*. The latter can grow on plain agar if staphylococci are added to supply the V factor. The V factor is also found in vegetables. In animal tissue and yeast, both X and V factors are present. Both factors are also present in blood, and they are liberated from the blood cells by heating. Levinthal (brain-heart infusion agar with heated and filtered blood) and chocolate agar are ideal media. *Haemophilus* species also grow on the usual blood agar. An atmosphere of carbon dioxide in a candle jar favors growth (Plate 18, Fig. 5). A great contribution was made by Pitman and Davis to the study of the differentiation of *H. aegyptius* and *H. influenzae*.

The colonies are tiny, glistening, translucent and pinpoint, with a dewdrop appearance (Plate 18, Fig. 4). The pronounced sweet odor is of great diagnostic aid and leads one to search for the tiny colonies which might easily be overlooked.

The satellite phenomenon, seen in the presence of staphylococcal colonies, especially *S. aureus,* is another important characteristic. (This phenomenon may also occur in the presence of other bacteria.) A zone of iridescent growth of bacilli is seen around a staphylococcal colony. Here the bacillary colonies are larger than the others on the plate (Plate 18, Fig. 4). Sometimes the presence of a single staphylococcal colony may make diagnosis possible, since the bacilli may grow only around that colony, the plate being otherwise barren.

Antigenic Structure. *H. aegyptius* and *H. influenzae* are closely related antigenically and are almost indistinguishable in other features.

The encapsulated forms of *H. influenzae* have specific polysaccharide antigens, which are related to the capsule and are responsible for the virulence of the organism. Since these bacilli easily lose their capsule, their antigenic property is not stable. The majority of antigenic types are found among the virulent S strains. Six antigenic types are distinguished, A to F. Serologically and chemically the bacillary capsular polysaccharides resemble those of the pneumococci, and serologic cross reaction with pneumococcal antigens is common. The Quellung test for the antigenic typing of *H. influenzae* is identical with the pneumococcal test.

Haemophilus bacilli can be identified by immunofluorescence or by specific rabbit antiserum (type B).

Pathogenesis. Although *H. influenzae* has produced infection in laboratory animals, *H. aegyptius* is not usually pathogenic for them. These bacilli do not produce endotoxin, and their mode of disease production is unclear.

The encapsulated *H. influenzae* is virulent, producing in man a suppurative inflammation mainly in the respiratory tract. The organism is not now regarded as the cause of influenza, but rather as a secondary invader to primary infection caused by the influenza virus. Nevertheless, there is still controversy concerning its role in influenzal diseases.

If the organism invades the blood, severe meningitis may develop in children under 3 years of age, with 98 percent mortality. In ophthalmology, acute conjunctivitis may precede the upper respiratory tract infection, which, on the other hand, may precede the meningitis. Therefore, conjunctivitis can be an indirect source of infection for meningitis. This relationship is critically important for both ophthalmologist and pediatrician.

It is known that in Egypt the trachomatous process was spread and aggravated by Koch-Weeks conjunctivitis (Haddad and McPhail). It could be true that the spread of upper respiratory tract infection, including viral, can be analogous with the above.

H. parainfluenzae emerged recently as pathogenic in a number of serious diseases, including ulcerative endocarditis and wound infections. In our study of 533 cases of *Haemophilus* eye infection, 102 were caused by *H. parainfluenzae,* an agent unknown before in ophthalmology.

Findings in the Eye. *H. aegyptius* is the principal etiologic agent for acute mucopurulent conjunctivitis, which occurs mainly in the summer, predominantly in southern climates (Minton). The exudate is mucoid in nature and not usually abundant. There is a great deal of associated lacrimation. The conjunctivitis becomes purulent if there is poor hygiene or low resistance. Clinically, it is similar to pneumococcal conjunctivitis and is characterized by involvement of the bulbar conjunctiva, which exhibits a typical cyanotic redness. Small hemorrhages may occur, mainly in the upper bulbar conjunctiva (Plate 18, Fig. 1), but these are not as prominent as they seem in pneumococcal conjunctivitis. Enlargement and tenderness of the preauricular glands occur. The bacilli are not easy to find in the secretion because of their small size and red color, which is hard to distinguish from the red background. A scraping from the bulbar conjunctiva may reveal the organism even prior to its appearance in the secretion. This infection is contagious and is usually epidemic, particularly in families, schools, or other institutions (Plate 18, Fig. 2).

The corneal involvement is unusual in our experience (Plate 18, Fig. 6). These bacilli have no affinity for corneal avascular tissue. However, in the tropics, corneal complications are not uncommon, and they may occur elsewhere. The author has described four cases of severe keratitis complicating acute conjunctivitis caused by *H. aegyptius*. This was observed in the 1927 epidemic of conjunctivitis at Dniepropetrovsk in the Ukraine. The cases of keratitis were perhaps a result of the greater virulence of the bacteria seen in this particular epidemic or of lowered resistance of these patients. Primary central corneal keratitis without preceding conjunctivitis is unknown.

Severe pseudomembranous conjunctivitis sometimes occurs in newborn children.

Cases of endophthalmitis caused by *H. aegyptius* have been occasionally recorded.

Haemophilus bacilli are not infrequently found in the pus from an infected lacrimal sac or in the secretion of the meibomian glands. Eleven cases of orbital cellulitis, caused by *Haemophilus*, in children 4 to 5 years old were reported recently (Londer and Nelson). These were correlated with anticapsular antibodies, and a high percentage of patients had a positive blood culture. The cellulitis was characterized by purple discoloration and a sharp border.

Treatment. The bacilli are susceptible to streptomycin, tetracyclines, and sulfonamides. Topical treatment suffices for the conjunctivitis. Most strains are sensitive to ampicillin and chloramphenicol. If there is a maternal lack of antibodies, immunization with capsular polysaccharides may be considered. The bacteriologic diagnosis and early treatment of *Haemophilus* conjunctivitis cannot be neglected.

Haemophilus ducreyi

This small gram-negative bacillus was described by Ducrey in 1889 as the cause of soft chancre (chancroid). The bacillus has many morphologic and biologic characteristics in common with *H. influenzae*. It has similar growth requirements, except that it needs only one of the growth factors, X, in the blood medium. Bacteriologic isolation of the bacillus from clinical material is very difficult, as it is usually associated with numerous other pyogenic bacteria.

For diagnosis of chancroid the skin test with killed culture of *H. ducreyi* bacilli is used. Ocular infections due to Ducrey's bacillus are extremely rare.

SMALL GRAM-NEGATIVE BACILLI

These are the smallest of all bacilli, having an imperfect inner structure. Hence, most of them are adapted to an intracellular habitat.

Laboratory identification is difficult, and strictly aseptic precautions are required because of high infectivity. Diagnosis is usually established by trained workers in specially equipped laboratories.

Bacilli of this group are rarely found in the eye. They are usually studied in detail by general bacteriologists. A few principal characteristics will be discussed briefly.

Brucella Genus

Members of this genus are classified according to their hosts: *Brucella melitensis* in goats, *Brucella abortus* in cattle, and *Brucella suis* in swine. The identification is not distinct, and they are sometimes considered variants of the same strain. All three, particularly *B. melitensis*, may cause brucellosis in man. *B. melitensis* was isolated from cases among military personnel on Malta, hence the popular name "Malta fever." It is septic in the acute stage, which becomes chronic, lasting for years. Milk and urine are the main sources of infection.

Man is highly susceptible to brucella, but the infection is frequently subclinical. The only positive diagnosis is the isolation of the organism from the blood or urine. Other tests, such as the skin test and agglutination tests, may be used as aids in the diagnosis but never in themselves assure it. Clinical manifestations are divided into three groups: acute, subacute, and chronic. The latter may last from 1 to 20 years.

Laboratory Studies. Brucella bacilli are found in direct secretion, are typically gram-negative, and are found within reticuloendothelial cells. Being tiny, the bacilli may be confused with intracellular granules.

Diagnosis is more successful with cultivation, but because of the intracellular habitat their nourishment requirements are complex. Some media require about 18 amino acids, vitamins, glucose, and salt.

Brucella bacilli grow on many media. *B. abortus* requires carbon dioxide tension, and Brewer's medium can be satisfactorily used. Identification of the species requires numerous additional factors.

Diagnosis is often made by ascertaining the agglutination titer of the patient's serum. Because the test is often positive in a healthy person, diagnosis of brucellosis should not be made unless the titer is at least 1:500. Usually titers of 1:60 and higher indicate infection. Recently, the presence of antibodies has been used for diagnosis. It was found that in the early stages, IgM antibodies are present, and later IgG. A titer of IgG of about 1:80 indicates active infection. Additionally the species can be differentiated by their individual sensitivity to dyes.

The patient's blood, or material from the lesions, or both, are used for laboratory investigation.

Findings in the Eye.   Brucellosis of the eye is secondary to systemic brucellosis, and primary invasion is almost unknown.

Involvements of the eye vary geographically (Cremona). They are rare, although in some countries they may be more frequent. When the eye is involved, the inner eye is predominantly affected, particularly the uvea. The process is usually the granulomatous type and may involve the entire uvea. In iritis, nodules occur at the pupillary border.

Nummular keratitis associated with brucellosis has been reported by Woods. He also produced this keratitis experimentally by inoculation with brucella, and has suggested the term "brucella nummular keratitis."

In Mexico, where brucellosis is widespread, the optic nerve is most frequently affected. Therefore, any patient with pathology of the optic nerve is routinely investigated for brucella.

Other ocular complications of systemic brucellosis are dacryocystitis and panophthalmitis, the latter appearing to be similar to that caused by the tubercle bacillus.

Treatment.   Chlortetracycline, chloramphenicol, oxytetracycline, and ampicillin give a striking result in treatment of brucellosis. Adding sulfadiazine and streptomycin may be helpful. Fever therapy is highly recommended. Vaccine therapy has been tried. Treatment is prolonged because of the intracellular habitat of the organisms.

Pasteurella, Yersinia, and *Francisella* Genera

These four bacilli, all associated with various animal hosts, were formerly grouped in the genus *Pasteurella*. The 8th edition of *Bergey's Manual* reclassifies three of these organisms into different genera. The species most affecting man are *Yersinia pestis, Yersinia pseudotuberculosis,* and *Francisella tularensis. Pasteurella multocida,* isolated from deer, is also pathogenic for man.

Y. *pestis* is a primary cause of disease in rats and various wild rodents. When transmitted to man it produces plague, which, without therapy, is invariably fatal. Sometimes the organisms are so highly virulent that a single bacillus can be lethal.

The bacilli are short, ovoid, plump, gram-negative rods. Many media are used to grow them, but blood agar plates are suitable for primary isolation. Ocular diseases due to Y. *pestis* are almost unknown.

Y. *pseudotuberculosis* produces disease in birds and various kinds of animals. Extremely rarely it may be transmitted to man.

F. *tularensis* is of interest in ophthalmology as a cause of Parinaud's oculoglandular syndrome. These bacilli are parasites of hares and wild rodents. The wild cottontail rabbit is the most common offender. It is transmitted by the bites of flies and tics. The name "tularemia" is from Tulare, a county in California where the disease was first identified. Tularemia can be transmitted to many by skinning or eating of animals infected with F. *tularensis*. Usually generalized and characterized by fever and adenopathy, the infection spreads via the blood to parenchymatous organs, and the disease may be fatal. Sometimes it is localized at the portal of entry, and it is usually associated with regional adenopathy. Transmission of infection among human beings is unknown.

Laboratory Studies. Morphologically, the bacilli are pleomorphic, tiny, usually coccobacillary, sometimes encapsulated, gram-negative.

F. *tularensis* does not grow on ordinary culture media. Egg yolk medium or blood glucose cystine agar is generally used for cultivation, and minute grayish white colonies develop. Brewer's medium, especially with fresh blood added, can also be satisfactorily employed, in a carbon dioxide atmosphere.

Specimens from local lesions or aspirated material from lymph nodes must be taken for smear culture and animal inoculation. Extreme precautions should be followed, since the material is highly contagious. Diagnosis of F. *tularensis* infection is a difficult problem, although much easier in time of epidemic.

Agglutination is a valuable diagnostic test for tularemia. The test is considered positive when agglutination occurs in serum diluted 1:80 or higher.

Findings in the Eye. The eye may be primarily affected through the conjunctiva, which is more vulnerable than is the skin, resulting in granulomatous conjunctivitis with possible ulceration. The incubation period is about three days, and the onset is sudden. The process is prolonged, about four weeks, is mainly unilateral, and is characterized by scattered, small, yellow, necrotic ulcers or nodules. The tarsal conjunctiva of the lower lid is primarily affected, although the upper lid can be involved. The infection is accompanied by fever and enlargement of the preauricular and submaxillary glands (oculoglandular Parinaud's syndrome). Suppuration of the glands, requiring an operation, is a frequent sequela. Nodular lesions resembling phlyctenules may occur rarely on the bulbar conjunctiva. This is characteristically painful. Although ocular tularemia is rare, 112 cases were reported in France in 1949–1950 (Brini and Muller; Rosenthal). These were predominantly the granulomatous type and were followed by ulceration. Systemic symptoms were usually absent, but Parinaud's syndrome was constantly present.

Treatment.   There is no specific treatment. The most effective is streptomycin and tetracycline. However, other broad-spectrum antibiotics may be effective in the early stages. A hot compress gives comfort.

ENTERIC BACTERIA

Hospital acquired, so-called nosocomial infections, are now a serious problem. The incidence of septicemia with a high mortality rate, particularly in surgery, and of upper respiratory tract infections has increased strikingly. About two-thirds of these infections are caused by gram-negative bacilli, particularly of the enteric group. There are increasing numbers of reports of serious infections due to many other gram-negative bacteria, so-called opportunists. This is associated with the wide use of broad-spectrum antibiotics, antimetabolic and suppressive therapy, and radiation, which disturb the balance of the normal flora, particularly regarding its beneficial symbiosis.

The enteric bacteria encompass a wide group of gram-negative bacilli, saprophytic and pathogenic, found in the intestinal canal. Although bacilli of the coliform group are a part of the normal flora, they may become pathogenic. The *Pseudomonas* and *Proteus* genera, related to the coliform group, are also discussed in this section.

The pathogens characteristically fail to ferment lactose. Hence, the lactose fermentation test is generally used as a preliminary one for differentiation of the enteric pathogens from nonpathogens.

The usually nonpathogenic enteric bacilli are not uncommon etiologic agents for infections of the genitourinary or respiratory tracts and of the eye or other parts of the body. They demonstrate pathogenicity if the host defense is low, as in infancy and old age, or if there is injured tissue. These bacilli have a number of common characteristics, a brief description of which may simplify diagnosis. All are morphologically indistinguishable, and their identification in smear is impossible. Culture is necessary. All are gram-negative bacilli, varying in size from short, coccobacillary forms to long filamentous ones, with rounded or pointed ends. Capsules are not constantly present except in the genus *Klebsiella*. There is nothing characteristic in the arrangement of the cells: they may be present singly, in pairs, in short chains, or in groups.

All members of this group grow readily on simple, ordinary media, even at room temperature. Colonies are semitranslucent and mucoid on solid media, with a tendency to become confluent. Many members are actively motile, and they all produce a strong odor. The species of all this group are differentiated by culture in media containing special dyes and carbohydrates.

They ferment a wide range of carbohydrates. Positive lactose fermentation differentiates most of these bacilli from the enteric pathogens, *Shigella* and *Salmonella*, which show negative lactose fermentation tests. Their complex antigenic structures result in serologic interrelationships among different groups and species.

Outside the intestinal canal these bacilli may produce a purulent type of inflammation, of which endotoxin is probably an important factor. Endotoxins injected in large doses into experimental animals produce hemorrhages and damage to the capillaries. They can elicit hemorrhagic necrosis of tumors and hemorrhages in utero, producing abortion.

Repeated daily injections of endotoxins result in tolerance, although endotoxins do not stimulate the production of antitoxins. The enteric bacilli are found often in normal flora of various mucosa or as secondary invaders because of the excessive use of antibiotics, which causes imbalanced flora. Their etiologic role can be determined only by repeated cultivation.

Coliform Bacteria

Escherichia coli, Enterobacter* aerogenes, and *Enterobacter* cloacae* are closely related, and their distinction is not easy, but it is particularly necessary for purposes of sanitation control. Finding *E. coli* in milk or water proves fecal contamination, but the presence of *Enterobacter* usually does not so indicate. Hence, may detailed differential tests have been devised to distinguish the organisms.

They exhibit some morphologic and cultural differences, eg, the capsule is more prominent and colonies are more mucoid in *E. aerogenes* than in *E. coli* (Plate 19, Fig. 1), but these are not constant characteristics and are not very significant. Biochemical characteristics are more important for differentiation. *E. coli* produces indole, the

*Formerly Aerobacter.

methyl red test is positive, the Voges-Proskauer test is negative, and there is no utilization of citrate. On the contrary, *Enterobacter* does not produce indole, the methyl red test is negative, and the Voges-Proskauer and citrate tests are positive. These differences may be demonstrated in the following media:

EMB (Eosin Methylene Blue) Agar. *E. coli* colonies are small and dry, with a characteristic green metallic sheen (Plate 19, Fig. 6). *Enterobacter* colonies are large, mucoid, and dark red in the center, though colorless on the periphery (Plate 19, Fig. 6).

MacConkey's Medium. *E. coli* colonies are usually large, dry, and bright pink (Plate 19, Fig. 2). *Enterobacter* colonies are moist and mucoid, and the center is usually red, with the periphery colorless.

Simmons' Citrate Agar. *E. coli* does not utilize citrate, and there is no color change in the medium. *Enterobacter* utilizes citrate and changes the medium from green to blue.

SIM Medium. *E. coli* is indole-positive; *Enterobacter* is indole-negative.

E. coli and *Enterobacter* show similarity in their pathogenicity and in their resistance to antibiotics. Hence in ophthalmology, distinct differentiation, which is rather complex, has more theoretical than practical interest.

Antigenic Structure. This is complex and varied in coliform organisms. *E. coli* has numerous flagellar, capsular, and somatic antigens. Two types of antigens are best known: O, a somatic antigen of the bacterial body, and H, a flagellar antigen. A capsular antigen, K, has been recognized. Most strains of *E. coli* are motile.

Pathogenicity and Pathology. Pathogenicity of *E. coli* is due to endotoxins and to the flagellar and capsular antigens. *E. coli* and, less frequently, *Enterobacter* may cause infections of the eye, gallbladder, the urinary or respiratory tracts, or elsewhere. *E. coli* in the newborn, particularly in the premature, causes urinary tract infection in epidemic form. The usual type of inflammation is purulent, with grayish green exudate. Any one of these infections can result in toxemia. Septicemia rarely develops in the newborn.

Findings in the Eye. *E. coli* seldom causes ocular infections (Berens and Nelson; Clark and Locatcher-Khorazo). It more often occurs as a secondary invader, and only repeated positive cultures can prove its causative role. It may be found in a small percentage of normal conjunctivas, especially in persons with intestinal ailments or following prolonged use of antibiotics.

In the conjunctiva, the bacillus has been described rarely as a cause of purulent ophthalmia in newborn infants. It may also cause pseudomembranous conjunctivitis in adults. Hypopvon keratitis due to

E. coli is uncommon, possibly because of a lack of affinity for corneal tissue (Vaughan). This severe hypopyon keratitis in the form of a deep abscess has been personally observed at Bellevue Hospital (Plate 19, Fig. 4). It is usually associated with corneal damage in debilitated patients.

The organism has also rarely caused panophthalmitis, cellulitis of the orbit, and dacryocystitis.

Treatment. The susceptibility of *E. coli* to antibiotics varies greatly, and sensitivity tests must be performed. The organisms may resist all antibiotics. Neomycin and polymyxin usually give a better result than do the other antibiotics. Sulfonamides, ampicillin, chloramphenicaol, and tetracycline can be effective. Wide-spectrum antibiotic treatment is more effective in severe cases, such as hypopyon keratitis. In our laboratory, sensitivity of *E. coli* to Kantrex has been demonstrated (Plate 19, Fig. 3). The pupil should be kept dilated in keratitis. If conjunctivitis alone is present, local treatment suffices.

Klebsiella Genus

This is a genus of coliform bacteria which, though closely related to *E. coli*, shows a more marked capsule and heavy mucoid growths. The organisms are classified mainly on the basis of the clinical picture. The varying nomenclature applied to *Klebsiella* in association with certain diseases is a source of confusion.

Klebsiella pneumoniae (Fiedeländer's bacillus) is found in patients with pneumonia. It is the most common respiratory pathogen causing hospital infection, which is characterized by necrotizing pneumonia. The clinical entities ozena and rhinoscleroma are possibly caused by *Klebsiella ozaenae* and *Klebsiella rhinoscleromatis*, respectively. The etiologic role of these bacilli is questioned, although they are found in the above diseases.

Calymmatobacterium (formerly *Donovania*) *granulomatis* shows a morphologic and antigenic resemblance to *Klebsiella*. It is the causative agent of granuloma inguinale, a venereal disease widespread in the tropics. The organism is found intracellularly in giant mononuclear cells and will grow in yolk sac.

Morphology. Morphologically *Klebsiella E. aerogenes* are distinguished from the other enteric bacilli by their heavy capsules, fat appearance, shortness (Plate 19, Fig. 1B), and the fact that they can occur as coccobacilli. The bacilli are a very faint pink with gram stain, although from an old culture they may not take the stain at all. The bacilli are arranged singly, in short chains, or as diplobacilli.

Culture. *Klebsiella* grow easily on simple media, as do all other enteric bacilli. They have a variety of cultural characteristics in association with the source of the culture. Nevertheless, the heavy mucoid appearance and a tendency to confluence are common and distinguishing characteristics of all *Klebsiella* and *Enterobacter* (Plate 19, Fig. 5). The mucoid consistency may be demonstrated by touching the colony with a loop; strings of material hang on the loop as it is removed. These organisms do not develop a characteristic odor and show no hemolysis. The culture is recognized usually without difficulty.

Klebsiella bacilli can be identified by the capsular swelling test.

Findings in the Eye.   *K. pneumoniae* may occur in the normal conjunctiva, but it is rarely the etiologic agent for a pathologic condition. However, a few ocular infections have been reported. These are keratitis in the form of a ring abscess, metastatic orbital abscess, dacryocystitis, pseudomembranous conjunctivitis of the newborn, even keratomalacia in infants. A pure culture of *K. pneumoniae* was isolated in our laboratory in a case of acute blepharoconjunctivitis.

The contact transference of the bacilli to the conjunctiva may occur sporadically in ozena. They may play a role in ocular infection, particularly of injured tissue. Their etiologic role can be decided only if the bacilli are plentiful in the conjunctival secretions, as they are usually secondary invaders.

Treatment.   The klebsiella bacilli are sensitive to most antibiotics except penicillin, and sensitivity tests help determine the choice. Since resistant strains appear rapidly, an antibiotic is best introduced together with sulfonamide, or two types of antibiotic should be used simultaneously.

Serratia Marcescens

Serratia marcescens, previously known as a nonpathogen, is now established as a causative agent of hospital nosocomial infection. *Serratia* septicemia, with a high mortality rate particularly postoperatively, has increased strikingly. *S. marcescens* has also been reported as causing meningitis, endophthalmitis, upper respiratory tract infection, and wound and burn infections. There are scattered reports of *Serratia* infection in ophthalmic literature.

Morphology.   *S. marcescens* are gram-negative bacilli of different sizes without characteristic arrangement, indistinguishable from the bacilli of the enteric group. In morphology from culture, coccal and coccobacillary forms are predominant.

Culture.   The bacilli grow easily even on ordinary media, as do all the enteric groups. The colonies are slightly mucoid, glistening, grayish, opaque centrally, and semitransparent at the periphery. Some strains of *Serratia* produce blood red pigment (Plate 20, Fig. 5). The test for identification is similar to that used for enterobacteria, but a positive DNAase test proves the diagnosis (Plate 20, Fig. 6). *Serratia* organisms ferment lactose very slowly.

Findings in the Eye. Postoperative endophthalmitis (Salceda et al), metastatic panophthalmitis (Bigger et al), purulent keratitis (Atlee et al), and conjunctivitis due to *S. marcescens* are known. In our experience severe metastatic panophthalmitis with ring abscess in a diabetic patient has been seen. Important contributing factors are diabetes, antibiotics particularly in their prophylactic use, cortisone, and the age of the patient (50 or over). However, there was a recent report of a corneal abscess in a healthy 9-year-old girl (Lazachek et al). *S. marcescens* infection may be associated with the use of contact lenses.

Treatment. *Serratia,* as well as all indigenous bacteria, are resistant to most antibiotics. Gentamycin and chloramphenicol can be used satisfactorily. The prognosis is usually serious.

Pseudomonas Genus

This is a broad group of bacilli distributed widely in soil and water.

Pseudomonas aeruginosa is a pathogen for man, and while saprophytic in the intestinal canal, it may become virulent outside.

In normal intestinal flora, *P. aeruginosa* multiplies rapidly if the coliform bacilli are suppressed, especially after prolonged treatment with antibiotics.

Pseudomonas is the cause of most severe postoperative infections and burn infections. It can be the cause of epidemic infection in the nursery.

It is reported to be the cause of postoperative infection, even sepsis, from contamination of solutions used in the operating room, eg, saline and others. The incidence of infection has greatly increased among wearers of contact lenses and in patients with lymphatic leukemia.

Morphologically, *P. aeruginosa* is indistinguishable from the other gram-negative enteric bacilli, and diagnosis in smear secretion is impossible (Plate 21, Fig. 1).

Culture. The culture, besides its general characteristics (p. 169), has a few distinguishing features. It produces two types of pigment: pyocyanin and fluorescein. Both pigments develop best at room temperature during daylight and in a fluid medium. In the latter, the pigment may best be demonstrated after shaking the tube to increase oxidation.

The colonies on blood agar are dark greenish gray, and because of pigment production the surrounding medium becomes bluish green (Plate 21, Fig. 2). Aged colonies have a gummy consistency, and vigorous scraping may be necessary to obtain a suitable specimen.

A strong, sweet, haylike odor is produced by *P. aeruginosa*.

On the basis of the cultural characteristics *P. aeruginosa* can usually be recognized without further testing.

For early diagnosis of *Pseudomonas* infection the Woods ultraviolet lamp has been used to demonstrate pyocyanin fluorescence. If there is sufficient pigment production, diagnosis can be made in situ.

It has recently been shown that *P. aeruginosa* may be highly bactericidal for other bacteria. This is possibly due to the lytic action of the pyocyanase or of the pigment.

Pathology.   *P. aeruginosa* was first isolated by Gessard in 1882 from "blue pus." The organism, outside the intestinal canal, is a common finding in the purulent inflammation of wounds, postoperative infections, and in the urinary tract. It is also found in infants' summer diarrhea and in inflammation of the middle and external ears. In the eye, *P. aeruginosa* causes the most destructive hypopyon keratitis.

Pseudomonas produces a variety of enzymes, including protease. In corneal destruction, both protease and collagenase play a role. It is believed that collagenase is produced not by bacteria but by damaged epithelial cells. It is the commonest cause of corneal ulcer in Central America. A septicemia complicated by endocarditis may occur. The bacilli cause patchy necrosis and ulceration on the skin. Nevertheless, in many of these conditions they may be only secondary invaders. *P. aeruginosa* has been isolated from the pharynx in cases of agranulocytic angina; however, the etiologic agent of the neutropenia is uncertain. The organism's pathogenicity may be proved in all these infections by inoculation of a culture into a rabbit cornea. If the organisms are virulent, an abscess develops.

P. aeruginosa is much more virulent in the tropics than in temperate regions and produces a systemic disease resembling typhoid fever.

Burns and Rhodes reported *Pseudomonas* infection as a cause of death in four premature infants.

Findings in the Eye.   Ocular disease due to *P. aeruginosa*, while uncommon, may be of great severity (MacDonald; Spencer).

A primary conjunctivitis seldom occurs, although purulent conjunctivitis, usually unilateral, may occur in the newborn. A membranous type of conjunctivitis, usually secondary to keratitis, has been reported (McCulloch). In our case of bilateral lacrimal mucocele, a pure culture of *P. aeruginosa* was isolated (Plate 21, Fig. 4).

Severe hypopyon keratitis may occur, which may be abscesslike (Plate 21, Fig. 3) or in the form of a ring abscess or ulcer (Bohigian and

Escapini; Golden et al; Hutton and Sexton; Okumoto et al, Williams et al). The process is characterized by a rapid course and necrosis, which may result in perforation within 24 hours. The only possibility of saving the eye is prompt recognition and early treatment. Signs and symptoms aiding early diagnosis follow:

1. There is nearly always a history of corneal injury, mostly by a foreign body.
2. In approximately 9 out of 10 cases there is a history of recent ocular therapy.
3. The chief ocular and early symptom is pain, occurring one to three days following the corneal insult. At the time, there are usually signs of corneal opacity and infiltration. Ulceration soon follows.
4. Epidemiology. The vast majority of cases appear in minor, sporadic epidemics which can usually be traced to a single source of contamination.

Summary.   To establish an early diagnosis, *P. aeruginosa* keratitis must be suspected in all cases that exhibit the following triad—(1) foreign body, (2) local therapy, and (3) ocular pain—one to three days after a corneal insult.

The eye infections ranged from conjunctivitis through corneal abscess to endophthalmitis, orbital cellulitis, and septicemia. Fisher and Allen showed in experiments that *P. aeruginosa* elaborates an enzyme, called protease, which has a proteolytic activity against collagen of the cornea. Therefore, the corneal process is rapid and necrotic. However, in all severe infections the host resistance is most important.

In ophthalmology, the ease and frequency with which fluorescein solution contaminated with *P. aeruginosa* created in the past a serious problem (Plate 21, Fig. 5). The obvious answer to the problem is the use of fluorescein strips. However, if the solution must be used, every precaution should be taken to ensure its sterility.

A dressing, particularly postoperatively, can create a favorable condition for the growth of *P. aeruginosa.*

Treatment.   Unfortunately, most antimicrobial agents have proved ineffective (Moorman and Harbert). However, the infection responds best to polymyxin B (Plate 21, Fig. 6). Colistin may help (Meleney et al), especially if administered early. An excellent result following prolonged therapy with subconjunctival polymyxin B in a dosage of 10 to 40 mg every two or three days has been reported. Gentamycin, a new drug, is said to be the best therapeutic agent thus far for *Pseudomonas* infection. Clinical observation is in process. In severe infection, shotgun therapy with antibiotics is advisable, with instillation of atropine to prevent iritis and posterior synechiae (Hessburg).

Prophylaxis. It is important to find and eliminate the source of contamination. All patients who have been exposed to the contaminant should receive local polymyxin therapy within three days. Rapid response may be obtained by antibiotics combined with steroids and enzymatic inhibitory therapy by injection beneath Tenon's capsule. Vaccination may help in severe burns, preventing sepsis.

Proteus Genus

The organisms of the *Proteus* genus have been known since the earliest days of bacteriology. *Proteus* bacilli, widely distributed in nature, exist as saprophytes in putrefying animal and vegetable matter. The bacilli rapidly decompose proteins and carbohydrates.

Proteus vulgaris, Proteus morganii, and *Proteus rettgeri* are of medical interest. *P. vulgaris* and *P. morganii* are usually saprophytic inhabitants of the intestinal canal. However, *P. morganii* has sometimes been a cause of summer diarrhea of children. Both may cause infection outside the canal.

Morphologically the organisms (Plate 20, Fig. 2) are indistinguishable from the other gram-negative bacilli.

Culture. Cultural characteristics of *Proteus* organisms are most significant for diagnosis. The ability of some to swarm on a solid medium, because of their active motility, is their most distinguishing feature. A uniform layer of spreading growth develops over the whole surface. The thin film is hard to see and may be overlooked, and scratching with a loop helps reveal the diffuse, filmy growth. The swarming growth often shows rippling waves moving either in one direction or in concentric rings, indicating periodic extensions of the growth (Plate 20, Fig. 3). *Proteus* bacilli produce a very strong odor of decay, easily detected at a distance. The bacilli may be recognized by these typical cultural characteristics. However, in atypical cases, several special tests are needed (Plate 20, Fig. 4). The positive urease test is most important.

Proteus bacilli frequently occur in mixed culture, swarming over the entire plate. They may mask the growth of organisms responsible for the infection. Therefore, narcotics, such as chloral hydrate or morphine, are used to inhibit spread of the *Proteus*.

Antigenic Structure. There are two main antigens, H (flagellar) produced by motile *Proteus,* and O (somatic) by nonmotile *Proteus.* Certain strains of *Proteus,* called X, have been isolated from the urine of patients with typhus fever, and the serum of the patient after four days agglutinated strains designated X19 and X2. Since the antigens are located in the bodies of nonmotile bacilli, they have been named OX19 and OX2. Agglutination of these strains by sera of patients with rickettsial infections is known as the Weil-Felix reaction. A positive Weil-Felix reaction has also been reported in trachoma.

Pathology. *Proteus* bacilli are usually found as secondary invaders in wounds. Nevertheless, they are responsible for several suppurative processes in man, such as urinary infection and cystitis. Numerous *Proteus* bacilli have been encountered in infantile diarrhea.

Findings in the Eye. *Proteus*, in the eye, is mainly a secondary contaminant. Since *Proteus* bacilli may be contaminants of the culture medium, it is absolutely necessary to repeat the culture several times. Only then can the etiologic role of *Proteus* be established.

Disease of the eye due to *P. vulgaris* is rare, although Crabb et al indicate that it has a higher pathogenicity for the eye than has been suggested (Okumoto et al, Smolin et al). *Proteus* has been isolated from cases of severe keratitis similar to those caused by *P. aeruginosa*. A similar case from Bellevue Hospital is shown in Plate 20, Fig. 1. The process is usually rapid and destructive and can result in perforation of the cornea. This keratitis most commonly occurs in older persons, after injury. Endophthalmitis caused by *Proteus* and panophthalmitis in premature infants have also been reported. Reports of postoperative endophthalmitis due to *Proteus mirabilis* or *P. morganii* have appeared (Peyman and Herbst). Diagnosis may be established by aspirated specimen. The disease is very severe, progresses rapidly, and is very stubborn to treatment.

Proteus bacilli are sometimes found in conjunctivitis, canaliculitis, dacryocystitis, in some postoperative infections, and in necrotic inflammation of the eyelid (Parunovic).

Treatment. The same problem is present as with other gram-negative bacilli. *Proteus* is the most stubborn and usually is not responsive to most antibiotics. In severe infections, shotgun therapy is recommended. Neomycin is the most active antibiotic. Streptomycin, chloromycetin, and neosporin have been successfully used. Ampicillin and gentamycin are the preferred drugs. The effect of rifampicin on *Proteus* keratitis has been studied experimentally and was shown to be as effective as gentamycin (Smolin and Okumoto).

CHLAMYDIA

The cause of psittacosis, lymphogranuloma venereum, trachoma, and inclusion conjunctivitis was considered to be large viruses for a long time because of their intracellular parasitism. Recently, it was discovered that their biologic characteristics are possibly related to gram-negative bacteria, which lack some important mechanism for the production of metabolic energy. These agents are classified in the 8th edition of *Bergey's Manual* as *Chlamydia,* a genus of Rickettsia. The two species are *Chlamydia trachomatis* and *Chlamydia psittaci. C. trachomatis* causes a variety of oculogenital diseases, including trachoma, inclusion conjunctivitis, and lymphogranuloma venereum. *C. psittaci* is the agent of several diseases, among them psittacosis and conjunctivitis.

The organisms are microscopic structures containing both nucleic acids, DNA and RNA, whereas viruses have only one. They form intracellular cytoplasmic inclusion bodies, which are enclosed in a matrix of protein or carbohydrate composition, showing a common morphologic cycle of intracellular development and possessing a considerable metabolism of their own. They do not grow on ordinary media and are inhibited by sulfonamides, as are bacteria. They also possess a bacterial wall.

The name TRIC was given by the Congress of Microbiology (Montreal, 1963) to the causative agent of Trachoma and Inclusion Conjunctivitis.

Psittacosis

Psittacosis was first reported in parrots; there were outbreaks in 12 states of the United States, in which the main pathology was pneumonia, with high mortality. From 1931 to 1956, 70 laboratory workers acquired the infection, with 7 known deaths. The parrot imported from South America was the source of infection (Meyer, Jawetz, 1960).

Acute follicular conjunctivitis with preauricular lymphadenopathy may develop in those who have parrots as pets, and the utmost care must be taken in handling parrots suspected of harboring *C. psittaci* (Schachter, Arnstein, Dawson et al). It is resistant to sulfonamides and most antibiotics but sensitive to tetracycline.

Lymphogranuloma Venereum

Lymphogranuloma venereum (LGV) is a disease common in the tropics and spread by venereal contact. *C. trachomatis* is the causative agent, according the 8th edition of *Bergey's Manual.* LGV is characterized by lesions on the genitalia, anus, and rectum and is accompanied by regional lymph node enlargement and systemic symptoms (Schachter). Ocular granular conjunctivitis may develop as a primary infection. Uveitis, keratouveitis, and sclerakeratitis of endogenous origin are known. Erythromycin and tetracycline are effective in treatment.

TRIC AGENTS

Lindner, in 1935, regarded the agents, then considered viruses, of trachoma and inclusion conjunctivitis to be identical. He believed that the TRIC agents were derived from the genitourinary tract and developed into trachoma agents by passage from eye to eye. There has been a considerable difference of opinion since that time as to whether the diseases are identical.

Trachoma had been distinguished from inclusion conjunctivitis by corneal involvement and scar formation. This concept has changed since Jones (1961; 1966) in London produced severe disease, with pannus and scarring, by inoculation of TRIC agents from conjunctivitis in the newborn into human volunteers. In addition, a trachoma agent inoculated into the genitourinary tract produced venereal disease, and specimens from cervicitis introduced into volunteers caused a conjunctivitis similar to trachoma. Jones believed that a maternal venereal infection is trachoma, and infant conjunctivitis is a neonatal form of trachoma. Hence Lindner's concept has been revived, and many contemporaries study this idea (Dawson and Schachter, 1967; Dunlop, Vaughan, Jackson, 1972; Thygeson, Hanna, Dawson, 1962).

Trachoma

Trachoma is a disease of the eye only, being local, without systemic involvement.

Trachoma affects about 400 million people in many lands and is still a major cause of blindness, although antibiotics have decreased the incidence to a significant degree.

In the Middle East, Africa, and the Orient, trachoma was once practically universal. In certain sections of the Balkans and Russia, a high incidence exists even now. Trachoma is uncommon in the United States, being localized mainly in some Indian reservations (Portney et al) of the Southwest and among the mountain people of Kentucky, Tennessee, and New Mexico. The incidence of active trachoma in the United States has been markedly reduced as a result of widespread improvement in environmental and social conditions. It flourishes where poor economic conditions and poor personal hygiene prevail. Young persons and children are more susceptible to trachoma than are adults, and mothers transfer the infection to their children. Trachoma can be spread by sharing of cosmetics. It is interesting that Blacks appear to be resistant to trachoma.

Clinical Features.   Great progress has been made in the laboratory study of trachoma. Early clinical diagnosis of trachoma is still most important.

Trachoma manifestations vary in different localities. In the United States the onset is usually acute. However, in a widespread personal experience in Russia, acute cases were rarely seen, and the onset was most frequently asymptomatic. Clinical surveys have revealed numerous cases in which the patient was unaware of this infection.

Early diagnosis is difficult because there are no pathognomonic symptoms until pannus or scarring develops (Dawson et al, 1967; Thygeson and Crocker). Initially, trachoma is characterized by follicles which are like follicles of other origin (Thygeson et al). While not morphologically different, the fact that these follicles predominate in the upper fornix and upper tarsal conjunctiva is significant (Plate 23, Fig. 2). The inflammatory infiltration of the surrounding conjunctiva is a cardinal differential sign. The conjunctiva lacks its usual transparency and appears red and thick, and the individual conjunctival vessels cannot be distinguished. A deep, penetrating subepithelial and tarsal inflammatory infiltration appears. As a result of the thickened conjunctiva and tarsus, trachomatous ptosis occurs (Plate 23, Fig. 4).

The discharge is generally mild unless bacterial infection ensues, when it can be abundant and purulent. In Egypt, *H. aegyptius* is constantly associated with trachoma, which causes the condition to appear similar to gonococcal conjunctivitis.

Corneal involvement is most important for early diagnosis. Collier et al, 1958 and Thygeson, 1962 emphasize the great importance of slit lamp examination. Limbal and corneal changes are invariably present in early trachoma, including vascularization of the limbus and epithelial keratitis. However, in some countries with endemic trachoma, pannus was absent in a high percentage of cases and was typical in adults. The slit lamp is not always available in trachomatous areas, and advanced pannus is often present at the initial examination. The upper cornea is the site of pannus involvement, which may relate to the predominant infection of the upper lid (Plate 23, Fig. 1). Constant contact of the cornea with a rough and thickened conjunctiva is worthy of consideration in the pathogenesis of the pannus. Mechanical rubbing, direct invasion by the agent, direct absorption of toxic or allergenic substances, and disturbances of nourishment by lid pressure must be considered as contributory factors.

The finding of characteristic inclusion bodies helps to confirm an early tentative diagnosis. In a later stage, follicles decrease in number.

Replacement by papillary hypertrophy and some cicatrization take place. The conjunctiva appears velvety and rough. Progressive infiltration of the tissues is noted. Simultaneously, the corneal process increases. According to its severity the pannus may be thin, tenuous, or very heavy (pannus crassus). The entire cornea may be involved, which is a leading cause of blindness (Plate 23, Fig. 5). All cases of pannus lead to corneal scarring.

The advancing margin of the pannus is often preceded by an unusually clear ulcer. Such ulcers cause corneal facets leading to decrease in vision because of changes in corneal refraction. Facets resulting from cicatrization of follicles occur at the limbus; these are so-called Herbert's pits. Bacterial infection frequently complicates the condition, with resultant severe purulent keratitis and subsequent blindness.

In later stages, various degrees of cicatrization develop (Plate 23, Fig. 3). The tissue infiltration and papillary hypertrophy decrease and finally disappear. A stage of pure cicatrization completes the process and results in lid deformation with trichiasis, entropion, or symblepharon. The heaviest scarring, causing incurving of the tarsus is found along the sulcus subtarsalis, an area rich in vessels. The corneal inflammation, while it may be found throughout the whole course of trachoma, usually becomes more mild or may even disappear in this stage. If in the cicatricial stage keratitis is found, it may be ascribed to the rubbing by the deformed lid.

The most tragic complication of trachoma is xerophthalmia, a type of cicatricial degeneration of the entire cornea and conjunctiva. These structures are dry, thick, and lusterless, resembling skin.

The division of trachoma into various stages is controversial. The following classification, which includes four stages, has been recommended for international use:

1. Incipient trachoma; onset of infection
2. Established trachoma
   A. Follicular hypertrophy predominant
   B. Papillary hypertrophy predominant
3. Cicatricial trachoma: appears simultaneously with remnants of inflammation
4. Healed trachoma: cicatricial

Laboratory Studies.   There were many attempts to grow the trachoma agent (*C. trachomatis*) and finally, in 1957, T'ang et al in China cultivated the trachoma agent in the yolk sac of embryonated eggs. This was confirmed by Collier and Sowa in England and Hanna et al (1960a) in the United States. Since that time, cultivation of *C. trachomatis* has been achieved in various parts of the world and confirmed by animal and volunteer inoculation (Collier et al; Dawson et al, 1962; Thygeson et al, 1935; Wang et al, 1967). There are described 19 or more isolated strains. The isolation of the trachoma agent in tissue culture has been achieved by Gordon et al and Furness et al (1960a), Collier, 1962.

The technique for isolation of the agents is basically the same as that described by T'ang. Using conjunctival scrapings, he made three positive isolations of the trachoma agent in the yolk sac of six-to eight-day old embryonated eggs. The material can also be taken from the conjunctiva by a swab wetted with 10 percent broth saline, and the best area for this is the upper tarsal conjunctiva. A heavy inoculum of the agent usually killed the embryos in 4 to 11 days. The egg-cultured agent produced a follicular conjunctivitis in rhesus monkeys and in volunteers.

Cultivation still presents difficulties. While developing the technique, it was noted that during certain seasons, the eggs were not susceptible to the trachoma agent. These were called "bad eggs," and according to Jawetz, the phenomenon occurs in the summer and usually lasts for one month. Variation in susceptibility was considered to be related to hormonal or nutritional disturbances among chickens. The presence of interferon can cause failure of growth. It is also important, for good growth, to use an early passage, the fourth passage being best (Jones). Bacterial contamination, particularly by staphylococci resistant to streptomycin, has complicated some studies.

The serologic data are not complete and need further clarification. Trachoma is a process without deep invasion or systemic involvement, hence, its immune response is poor. It was felt for a long time that no antibody formation or increase of host resistance occurred during active trachoma infection. Serologic studies have been accelerated by the recent advances in cultivation of the trachoma agent. There are already at least nine antigenic types of TRIC agents (A to I). There is some evidence that antibodies may affect the course of infection. Woolridge and Grayston purified antigens for study in complement-fixation tests, and they detected antibodies (Hanna et al, 1973; Wang, McComb, 1974) in sera of trachomatous patients. Antibodies are produced regularly by the infected host but they have little protective effect.* The prevention of trachoma by vaccination has been studied by many others (Bietti, Scott).

The study of inclusion bodies has a long history, but little has been added. The inclusion bodies of trachoma and of inclusion conjunctivitis, known as Halberstädter-Prowazek bodies, are morphologically

---

*The infection may persist in the presence of a high titer of antibodies.

indistinguishable (Plate 22, Fig. 1). They are basophilic, epithelial, and cytoplasmic, being aggregations of granules, usually in the form of a cap, which appears to grasp the nucleus and may even partially occupy it. Occasionally more than one inclusion body is found in a cell. The inclusion bodies represent colonies of elementary bodies and a few initial bodies.

The development cycle of the inclusions was established by Bedson and by Thygeson et al, 1935 as follows: the infectious unit is an elementary body which has a core of DNA, RNA, and a coat of protein. These are small, regular in size, purple (with Giemsa stain) particles, which infect the cell by the process of phagocytosis. As a result of biosynthesis with the cells, the elementary bodies reorganize into large initial bodies which are mildly infected particles. Initial bodies are divided by binary fission, as are bacteria, into elementary bodies. The conglomerate of all these particles is called an "inclusion body" and is enveloped in a capsule, which may occupy the entire cytoplasm. The main mass is composed of elementary bodies. Among these are scattered a few large initial bodies of different shape and blue in color (Giemsa stain) (Plate 22, Fig. 1). Lugol's iodine has been used to demonstrate a glycogenic matrix which surrounds the particles and stains brown (Thygeson, 1938).

When a cell ruptures, the elementary body is liberated and invades other epithelial cells. The study of the cytology of the scrapings is an additional important diagnostic method (Plate 22, Figs. 1, 4).

The most sensitive method for diagnosis is immunofluorescence (Wang, Grayston, 1974). However, isolation of the organism determines the diagnosis.

The finding of inclusion bodies is significant for early diagnosis of trachoma and for differentiation from other conjunctival processes. Their identification is not always simple, as they can be easily confused with other granules or, frequently, with pigment of varied origin, especially the melanin of dark-skinned patients. The pigment granules are distinguished by their irregular size, shape, and differing color, being green, brown, or very dark blue. They have no specific arrangement. Epithelial cells containing inclusion bodies are usually larger than normal, while those with pigment granules are of normal size (Plate 22, Fig. 2).

In the early stage of trachoma, inclusion bodies are usually numerous and readily demonstrated in scrapings from the upper tarsal conjunctiva (Braley, 1939).

Leber cells, while not specific, provide a possible clue for diagnosis (Plate 22, Fig. 4). The author has demonstrated Leber cells in material expressed from ripe follicles of folliculosis. These are giant histiocytic macrophages, or cells of epithelial origin, showing well-marked nucleoli. Lymphocytes and often lymphoblasts (Biantovskaya and Shapiro) and plasma cells predominate in the scraping, and monocytes are also common (Plate 44, Figs. 1–3). In the acute stage, neutrophils predominate. Vacuolized cells, the shadow cells of Humprecht, and tissue debris are additional findings in trachoma scrapings.

Trachoma is best studied in sections of tarsus with subepithelial tissue (Plate 22, Fig. 3). Excision of the heavily involved tarsus is still an approved form of treatment. In the trachomatous area, partial or complete incision of the thickly infiltrated tarsus is the popular method of treatment. In section, heavy diffuse infiltration with lymphocytes, plasma cells, and, very rarely, follicles are found. This occurs mainly along the upper and lower arterial arches (perivascular exudation). The development of fibrous tissue in the late stage is a distinct feature.

Electron microscopy of trachoma virus in section have been done by Mitsui and Suzuki. Some observers feel that trachoma is not a single inflammatory process but a lymphoid hyperplasia.

Trachoma is a contagious disease transmitted from eye to eye. The incubation period is uncertain, since subclinical infection is the rule. Its latency, even after treatment, can last a lifetime and relapses occur. The incubation period for inclusion conjunctivitis in experimental work is 14 to 48 hours, and in the newborn 5 to 12 days.

The related bacterial conjunctivitis or any kind of irritants may exacerbate the process. It is known that in Egypt in the endemic area, many children developed trachoma after an attack of *H. aegyptius* conjunctivitis or other bacterial infection (Haddad, McPhaill). These organisms spread and aggravate the trachomatous process and may stimulate the silent trachoma. Flies play the most important role in spreading of infection.

Treatment. Coppersulfate (bluestone) was used in former times, often year after year. This is now condemned, for it may create more damage than the disease itself.

Tetracycline and erythromycin can be the most effective topical antibiotics for trachoma (Dawson et al, 1974). Treatment two to four times daily should be continued for at least three months. Sulfonamides have been given orally, but there are opinions that they do not appear to be more effective than topical antibiotics. Vaccination in an endemic area has often given promising results (Bietti et al; Thygeson, Scott, 1971).

In the cicatricial sequel, surgical treatment is indicated. Many different operations are used. Mucous membrane grafts from the lip into the intermarginal space is an excellent approach in trichiasis. When the tarsus is heavily thickened, its partial or entire excision (Kuhnt procedure) has had a recognized success.

If the cornea is involved, routine treatment for keratitis must be added.

Proper nutrition and personal hygiene are important in inhibiting the spread of trachoma.

Certain social conditions must be considered in the spread of trachoma. Poverty, poor nutrition, neglect of public as well as personal hygiene, and overcrowding are factors decreasing resistance and favoring dissemination of the infection.

Inclusion Conjunctivitis (Oculogenital Diseases)

Two age clinical entities may be distinguished: inclusion conjunctivitis of the newborn and inclusion conjunctivitis of adults.

Inclusion Conjunctivitis of Newborn. This is an acute, purulent conjunctivitis occurring 5 to 10 days after birth. The infant is infected as it passes through the birth canal. The process is characterized by a profuse purulent exudate (Plate 24, Fig. 1). It may begin bilaterally or unilaterally, in which case the second eye is usually involved 3 to 7 days later. The lower lid is more severely involved than the upper. Papillary hypertrophy is not uncommon, and in severe cases, pseudomembrane formation can be seen. The process is self-limited, with complete healing in 10 to 12 days. Chronic cases are usually rare, and the cornea is usually uninvolved. However, differentiation from trachoma on the basis of corneal involvement is not supported by some contemporary studies. Different kinds of superficial keratitis, including pannus and scarring, have been observed (Dawson et al, 1967; Thygeson and Dawson, 1966). Eye-to-eye contamination is very rare. The infection is commonly limited to a single member of a family.

The disease must be differentiated from gonococcal conjunctivitis of the newborn. The short incubation period for the gonococcus, 2 to 3 days, and the laboratory finding of gonococci are important for diagnosis.

Inclusion Conjunctivitis of Adults. This is an acute follicular conjunctivitis. The disease is caused by the same agent as is inclusion conjunctivitis of infants but has several different clinical features. The discharge is scanty in adults. There is more roughness and redness of the conjunctiva with follicles and papillary formation (Plate 24, Fig. 2), and the preauricular nodes are enlarged (in the newborn this is absent). The process is usually unilateral, of long duration, sometimes lasting years, and mildly contagious. Poorly chlorinated swimming pools, infected from the genitourinary tract, are a source of infection. Typical inclusion bodies differentiate this condition from other forms of follicular conjunctivitis, with the exception of trachoma.

Reiter's syndrome and otitis media have been associated with inclusion conjunctivitis (Dawson et al, 1970; Mohsenine and Dorougar).

Laboratory Studies. This question has been discussed on page 174. Numerous investigators have worked in this area, and especially significant contributions has been made by Allen, Braley, Julienelle (Thygeson), and others.

However, attempts to cultivate the inclusion conjunctivitis agent failed. Only in 1959 was its isolation reported by Jones, Collier, and Smith. They employed the same technique as had been used for isolation of the trachoma agent in the yolks of embryonated eggs. Two isolations were made: one from inclusion conjunctivitis, the other from the cervix. Jones and Collier later established that a strain present in the female genital tract, introduced from the resultant neonatal conjunctivitis, is capable of producing the picture of trachoma in the adult eye. The first isolation in the United States of the inclusion conjunctivitis agent was reported in 1960a by Hanna et al. Later, its successful growth in cell culture was reported (Collier, 1962; Furness et al, 1960a; Gordon). Recently Thygeson et al achieved positive inoculation of human volunteers with egg-grown inclusion conjunctivis agent (1962).

Although *C. trachomatis* is the etiologic agent of both inclusion conjunctivitis and trachoma, the clinical manifestations and epidemiology of the two diseases are different.

Isolation of *C. trachomatis* and purification and concentration techniques in the yolks of embryonated eggs greatly accelerated studies of its serology and immunity.

Cytologic features are the same in the scrapings from both clinical entities of inclusion conjunctivitis. Inclusion bodies, indistinguishable from those of trachoma, are most significant for diagnosis. Contrary to the site in trachoma, they are usually found in scrapings from the lower lid. Predominant neutrophilic and monocytic responses are additional differential characteristics. Monocytes are usually markedly vacuolized (Plate 24, Fig. 3).

Treatment. Treatment is not a problem in the newborn, as the condition is self-limited. The process responds readily to local treatment with sulfonamides; additionally, tetracycline may be effective. In adults, local treatment with the previously mentioned drugs, plus systemic or oral sulfonamide treatment if the condition does not respond, may be needed to prevent a chronic course.

REFERENCES

Bacterial Morphology, Host-Parasite Relationships

Allansmith MR, Hahn G, Simon M: Tissue tear and serum IgE concentrations in vernal conjunctivitis. Am J Ophthalmol 81:506, 1976a

Allansmith MR, Kajiyama G, Abelson M, Simon M: Plasma cells in lacrimal glands. Am J Ophthalmol 82:819, 1976b

Allansmith MR, Whitney CR, McClellan BH, Newman LP: Immunoglobulins in the human eye. Arch Ophthalmol 89:36, 1973

Aronson SB, Goodner EK, Yamamoto E, Foreman M: Mechanisms of the host response in the eye. Arch Ophthalmol 73:402, 1965

Brown S, Mondino B, Rabin B: Autoimmune phenomenon. Am J Ophthalmol 82:835, 1976

Cason L, Winkler CH Jr: Bacteriology of the eyes. I. Normal flora. Arch Ophthalmol 51:196, 1954

Kaufman HE, Brown DC, Ellison ED: Herpes virus in the lacrimal gland, conjunctiva and cornea: a chronic infection. Am J Ophthalmol 65:32, 1968

Leopold J: The 1975 Bedell lecture: Clinical immunology in ophthalmology. Am J Ophthalmol 81:129, 1976

Savage D, Cogan G, Nienhuis A, Mina J: Conjunctival infiltration by plasma cells. Am J Ophthalmol 82:486, 1976

Silverstein AM: The immunologic modulation of infectious disease pathogenesis. Invest Ophthalmol 13:560, 1974

Theodore FH, Schlossman A: Ocular Allergy. Baltimore, Williams & Wilkins, 1958

Thygeson P: Marginal corneal infiltrates and ulcers. Arch Ophthalmol 39:432, 1948

Thygeson P: The cytology of conjunctival exudates. Am J Ophthalmol 29:1499, 1946

Weeks JE: The bacillus of acute conjunctival catarrh or pink eye. Arch Ophthalmol 15:441, 1886

Winkler CH Jr, Cason L: Bacteriology of the eyes. II. Role of gram-negative bacilli infections following cataract extraction. Arch Ophthalmol 51:200, 1954

Woods AC: The diagnosis and treatment of ocular allergy. Am J Ophthalmol 32:1457, 1949

Gram-positive Group, Mycobacteria

Allen JH: Experimental production of conjunctivitis with staphylococci. Am J Ophthalmol 22:1218, 1939

Allen JH, Byers JL: The pathology of ocular leprosy. 1. The cornea. Arch Ophthalmol 64:216, 1960

Baker TR, Spencer WH: Ocular findings in multiple myeloma. Arch Ophthalmol 91:110, 1974

Baum J, Rao G: Keratomalacia. Am J Ophthalmol 82:435, 1976

Berens C, Nilson EL: Relationship between the bacteriology of the conjunctiva and nasal mucosa. Am J Ophthalmol 27:747, 1944

Brown JH: The use of blood agar for the study of streptococci. The Rockefeller Institute for Medical Research (Monograph 9), 1919, 122 pp

Buchanan RE, Gibbons NE (eds): Bergey's Manual of Determinative Bacteriology, 8th ed. Baltimore, Williams & Wilkins, 1974

Burns RP: Postoperative infections in an ophthalmic hospital. Am J Ophthalmol 48:519, 1959

Chace RR, Locatcher-Khorazo D: Keratoconjunctivitis due to a diphtheroid-like organism. Arch Ophthalmol 37:497, 1947

Darrel RW: Acute tuberculous panophthalmitis. Arch Ophthalmol 78:51, 1967

Davenport R, Smith C: Panophthalmitis due to an organism of the *Bacillus subtilis* group. Br J Ophthalmol 36:389, 1952

Elliot DC: Leprosy, a disease of childhood: with special reference to early findings in the eye, ear, nose and throat of children examined at the national leprosorium at Carville, Louisiana. J Pediatr 35:189, 1949

Fritz MH, Thygeson P, Durham DG: Phlyctenular keratoconjunctivitis among Alaskan natives. Am J Ophthalmol 34:177, 1951

Harley RD: Ocular leprosy in Panama. Am J Ophthalmol 29:295, 1946

Henkind P, Fedukowicz H: Clostridium welchii conjunctivitis. Arch Ophthalmol 70:791, 1963

Jawetz E, Melnick JL, Adelberg EA: Review of Medical Microbiology, 5th ed. Los Altos, Cal, Lange Medical Publications, 1962; 9th ed., 1970

Johnson MK, Allen JH: The role of cytolysin in pneumococcal ocular infection. Am J Ophthalmol 80:518, 1975

Johnson MK, Allen JH: Ocular toxin of the pneumococcus. Am J Ophthalmol 72:175, 1971

Joklik WK, Willet HP: Zinsser Microbiology, 16th ed. New York, Appleton, 1976, p 495

Julianelle LA, Boots RH, Harrison GH: The treatment of staphylococcal infections of the eye by immunization with toxoid. Am J Ophthalmol 25:431, 1942

Kennedy PJ: Ocular manifestations in leprosy. Am J Ophthalmol 35:1360, 1952

König H, Gassman H, Jenzer G: Ocular involvement in benign botulism, Am J J Ophthalmol 80:430, 1975

Krauss F, Spikes NO: Edematous anthrax of the face resulting in meningitis. Am J Ophthalmol 9:337, 1926

Lancefield RC: A serological differentiation of human and other groups of hemolytic streptococci. J Exp Med 57:571, 1933

Lauring LM, Wergeland FL, Sack GE: Anonymous mycobacterium keratitis. Am J Ophthalmol 67:130, 1969

Leavelle RB: Gas gangrene panophthalmitis. Arch Ophthalmol 53:634, 1955

Locatcher-Khorazo D, Gutierrez E: Bacteriophage typing of *Staphylococcus aureus*. Arch Ophthalmol 63:774, 1960

Macoul KL: Pneumococcal septicemia presenting as hypopyon. Arch Ophthalmol 81:144, 1969

McEntyre JM, Curran KE: Gas gangrene panophthalmitis. Am J Ophthalmol 65:109, 1968

Okumoto M, Smolin G: Pneumococcal infections of the eye. Arch Ophthalmol 77:346, 1974

Ostler H, Okumoto M: Anaerobic streptococcal corneal ulcer. Am J Ophthalmol 81:518, 1976

Pasteur L: Bull Acad Nat Med (2me série):76, 1881

Pendergast JJ: Ocular leprosy in the United States. Arch Ophthalmol 23:112, 1940

Rhodes AJ: Studies on the bacteriology of hypopyon ulcer. Br J Ophthalmol 23:627, 1939

Richards WW, Arrington JN: Unsuspected ocular leprosy. Am J Ophthalmol 68:492, 1969

Scobee RG: The role of the meibomian glands in recurrent conjunctivitis. Am J Ophthalmol 25:184, 1942

Shepard CC: The experimental disease that follows the injection of human leprosy bacilli into foot pads of mice. J Exp Med 112:445, 1960

Spaeth GL: Chronic membranous conjunctivitis. Am J Ophthalmol 64:300, 1961

Suie T, Taylor FW: Incidence of coagulase-positive staphylococci in external ocular infections. Arch Ophthalmol 53:706, 1955

Theodore FH, Schlossman A: Ocular Allergy. Baltimore, Williams & Wilkins, 1958

Theodore FH, Schlossman A: "Silent" dacryocystitis. Arch Ophthalmol 40:157, 1948

Thygeson P: Observations on non-tuberculous phlyctenular keratoconjunctivitis. Trans Am Acad Ophthalmol 58:128, 1954

Thygeson P: Treatment of staphylococcic blepharoconjunctivitis with staphylococcus toxoid. Arch Ophthalmol 26:430, 1941

Touren S, Cornet P, Midy C, Pettiss S: Xerophthalmia and blindness. Am J Ophthalmol 82:439, 1976

Trantas M: Keratite ponctuee lepreuse. Arch Ophthalmol 32:193, 1912

Tsutsui J: Tetanus infection of the cornea. Am J Ophthalmol 43:772, 1957

Valenton MJ, Okumoto M: Toxin-producing strains of *Staphylococcus epidermidis*. Arch Ophthalmol 89:187, 1973

Vaughan DG Jr: Corneal ulcers. Surv Ophthalmol 43:772, 1957

Weeks JE: Tuberculosis of the eye. Am J Ophthalmol 9:243, 1926

Weiss C, Shevky MC, Perry IH: Experimental investigation of the pathogenicity of diphtheroids isolated from the human conjunctiva. Arch Ophthalmol 40:23, 1948

Wilson GS, Miles AA: Topley and Wilson's Principles of Bacteriology and Immunity, 4th ed. Baltimore, Williams & Wilkins, 1955

Zimmerman LE, Turner L, McTigue JW: *Mycobacterium fortuitum* infection of the cornea: a report of two cases. Arch Ophthalmol 82:596, 1969

Gram-negative Group

Allen JH, Erdman GL: Meningococcic keratoconjunctivitis. Am J Ophthalmol 29:721, 1946

Atlee WE, Burns RP, Oden M: *Serratia marcescens* keratoconjunctivitis. Am J Ophthalmol 70:31, 1970

Axenfeld T: Uber die chronische Diplobacillenconjunctivitis. Zentralbl Bakteriol 21:1, 1897

Baraff AAA: Gonorrheal ophthalmia neonatorum. Ill Med J 87:249, 1945

Berens C, Nilson EL: Ocular conditions associated with coliform bacteria. Arch Ophthalmol 26:816, 1941

Bigger JF, Meltzer G, Mandel A, et al: *Serratia marcescens* endophthalmitis. Am J Ophthalmol 72:1102, 1971

Bohigian GM, Escapini H: Corneal ulcer due to *Pseudomonas aeruginosa*. Arch Ophthalmol 85:405, 1971

Brini A, Muller J: Oculo-glandular tularemia and the conjunctivitis of Parinaud (abstract). Am J Ophthalmol 35:159, 1952

Buchanan RE, Gibbons NE (eds): Bergey's Manual of Determinative Bacteriology, 8th ed. Baltimore, Williams & Wilkins, 1974

Burns RP, Rhodes DM: Pseudomonas eye infection as a cause of death in premature infants. Arch Ophthalmol 65:517, 1961

Clark G, Locatcher-Khorazo D: Corneal ulcer produced by *Aerobacter aerogenes*. Arch Ophthalmol 45:165, 1951

Crabb AM, Fielding IL, Ormsby HL: *Bacillus proteus* endophthalmitis. Am J Ophthalmol 43:86, 1957

Cremona AC: Ocular manifestations of human brucellosis (abstract). Am J Ophthalmol 37:320, 1954

deBord GG: Descriptions of Mimeae tribe with three genera and three species and two new species of *Neisseria* from conjunctivitis and vaginitis. Iowa St Coll J Sci 16:471, 1942

Fedukowicz H, Alterman M, Newman R: Two decades of experience with Moraxella. Exerpt Med Internat Congress Ophthalmol Series 22, March 1970

Fedukowicz H, Horwich H: The gram-negative diplobacillus in hypopyon keratitis. Arch Ophthalmol 40:202, 1953

Feldman M: The Koch-Weeks bacillus and John Weeks. Arch Ophthalmol 70:430, 1963

Fisher E Jr, Allen JH: Mechanisms of corneal destruction by pseudomonas proteases. Am J Ophthalmol 46 (Part 2):249, 1958

Fox JE, Lowbury EJL: Immunity to *Pseudomonas pyocyanea* in man. J Pathol Bacteriol 65:519, 1953

Givner I: *Neisseria catarrhalis* endophthalmitis. Am J Ophthalmol 32:699, 1949

Golden B, Fingerman LH, Allen HF: *Pseudomonas* corneal ulcers in contact lens wearers. Arch Ophthalmol 85:543, 1971

Haddad NA, McPhail JJ: Mucopurulent conjunctivitis and haemophilus. Am J Ophthalmol 68:35, 1969

Henriksen SD: Moraxella, classification and taxonomy. J Gen Bacteriol 6:318, 1952

Hessburg PC: Treatment of *Pseudomonas* keratoconjunctivitis in humans. Am J Ophthalmol 61:896, 1966

Horwich H, Fedukowicz H: Variation in Morax-Axenfeld diplobacillus. Arch Ophthalmol 54:580, 1955

Hutton WL, Sexton RR: Atypical *Pseudomonas* corneal ulcers in semicomatose patients. Am J Ophthalmol 73:37, 1972

Jensen AD, Naidoff MA: Bilateral meningococcal endophthalmitis. Arch Ophthalmol 90:396, 1973

Kahaner JR, Lanou WW: Exogenous meningococcic conjunctivitis. NY J Med 45:1687, 1945

King EO: Mimeae infections. In Diagnostic Procedures and Reagents, 4th ed. New York, American Public Health Assoc, 1964, Chap 22

Koch R: II. Bericht über die thätigkeit der deutschen Cholerakomission in Aegypten und Ostindien. Wien Med Wochenschr 33:1548, 1883

Lazachek GW, Boyle GL, Schwartz AL, et al: *Serratia marcescens*: an ocular pathogen. Arch Ophthalmol 86:599, 1971

Londer L, Nelson DL: Orbital cellulitis due to *Haemophilus influenzae*. Arch Ophthalmol 91:89, 1974

MacDonald M: *Ps. pyocyaneus* eye infection. Br J Ophthalmol 37:370, 1953

Mangiaracine AB, Pollen A: Meningococcic conjunctivitis. Arch Ophthalmol 31:284, 1944

McCulloch JC: Origin and pathogenicity of *Pseudomonas pyocyanea* in conjunctival sac. Arch Ophthalmol 29:924, 1943

Meleney FL, Prout GR Jr: Some laboratory and clinical observations on Colymycin (Colistin) with particular reference to pseudomonas infection. Surv Ophthalmol 6:433, 1961

Minton J: Eye diseases in the East. Br J Ophthalmol 29:19, 1945

Mitsui Y, Hinokuma S, Tanaka C: Etiology of angular conjunctivitis. Am J Ophthalmol 34:1579, 1951

Mondino B, Kessler E, Gipson L, Brown S: Effect of zinc sulfate on pseudomonas aeruginosa infections and protease in rabbit corneas. Arch Ophthalmol 94:2149, 1976

Moorman LT, Harbert F: Treatment of Pseudomonas corneal ulcers. Arch Ophthalmol 53:345, 1955

Odegaard K: Conjunctivitis purulenta with keratitis caused by *Neisseria intracellularis*. Acta Ophthalmol 21:295, 1944

Oeding P: *Diplobacillus liquefaciens* of Petit isolated from a patient with ulcus serpens corneae. Acta Ophthalmol 24:159, 1946

Okumoto M, Smolin G, Belford R, Kim H, Siverio C: Proteus species isolated from human eyes. Am J Ophthalmol 81:495, 1976

Parunovic A: *Proteus mirabilis* causing necrotic inflammation of the eyelid. Am J Ophthalmol 76:543, 1973

Peyman GA, Herbst R: Bacterial endophthalmitis. Arch Ophthalmol 91:416, 1974

Presley GD, Hale LM: Corneal ulcers due to *Bacterium anitratum*. Am J Ophthalmol 65:571, 1968

Reid RD, Bronstein LH: Meningococcic conjunctivitis. JAMA 124:703, 1944

Rosenthal JN: Oculoglandular tularemia (abstract). Am J Ophthalmol 34:163, 1951

Salceda SR, Lapuz J, Vizconde R, et al: *Serratia marcescens* endophthalmitis. Arch Ophthalmol 89:163, 1973

Shore WB, Winkelstein JA: Non-venereal transmission of gonococcal infections to children. J Pediatr 79:661, 1971

Smolin G: Proteus endophthalmitis. Arch Ophthalmol 91:419, 1974

Smolin G, Okumoto M: Effect of rifampicin on proteus keratitis. Am J Ophthalmol 73:40, 1972

Spaeth GL: Treatment of penicillin-resistant gonococcal conjunctivitis with ampicillin. Am J Ophthalmol 66:427, 1968

Spencer WH: *Pseudomonas aeruginosa* infections of the eye. Calif Med 79:438, 1953

Theodore FH: The classification and treatment of allergies of the conjunctiva. Am J Ophthalmol 36:1689, 1953

Theodore FH, Kost PF: Meningococcic conjunctivitis. Arch Ophthalmol 31:245, 1944

Thygeson P, Kimura S: Chronic conjunctivitis. Trans Am Acad Ophthalmol Otolaryngol 67:494, 1964

van Bijsterveld OP: Host-parasite relationship and taxonomic position of Moraxella and morphologically related organisms. Am J Ophthalmol 76:545, 1973

van Bijsterveld OP: The incidence of Moraxella on mucous membranes and skin. Am J Ophthalmol 74:46, 1972

van Bijsterveld OP: Bacterial proteases in Moraxella angular conjunctivitis. Am J Ophthalmol 72:181, 1971

Vaughan DG Jr: Corneal ulcers. Surv Ophthalmol 3:203, 1958

Wand M, Olive GM, Mangiaracine AB: Corneal perforation and iris prolapse due to *Mima polymorpha*. Arch Ophthalmol 93:239, 1975

Weeks JE: The bacillus of acute conjunctival catarrh or "pink eye." Arch Ophthalmol 15:441, 1886

Williams RK, Hench ME, Guerry DuP: III. Pyocyaneus ulcer. Am J Ophthalmol 37:538, 1954

Woods AC: Nummular keratitis and ocular brucellosis. Arch Ophthalmol 35:490, 1946

Chlamydia

Allen JH: Inclusion blennorrhea. Am J Ophthalmol 27:833, 1944

Bedson SP: Observation on the developmental forms of psittacosis virus. Br J Exp Pathol 14:267, 1933

Biantovskaya (Fedukowicz) ET, Shapiro EI: Diagnostic significance of cytologic examination of follicles of adenoid tissue in trachoma. Sov Vestnik Oftal 4:596, 1934

Bietti GB, Werner GH: Results of large-scale vaccination against trachoma. Am J Ophthalmol 61:1010, 1966

Braley AE: The relation between the virus of trachoma and the virus of inclusion blennorrhea. Arch Ophthalmol 22:393, 1939

Buchanan RE, Gibbons NE (eds): Bergey's Manual of Determinative Bacteriology, 8th ed. Baltimore, Williams & Wilkins, 1974

Collier LH: Growth characteristics of inclusion blennorrhea virus in cell cultures. Ann NY Acad Sci 98:42, 1962

Collier LH, Duke-Elder WS, Jones BR: Experimental trachoma produced by cultured virus. Br J Ophthalmol 42:705, 1958

Collier LH, Sowa J: Isolation of trachoma virus in embryonate eggs. Lancet, 1:993, 1958

Dawson CR, Daghfous MD, Messadi M, et al: Severe endemic trachoma in Tunisia. A control therapy trial of topically applied chlortetracycline and erythromycin. Arch Ophthalmol 92:198, 1974

Dawson CR, Mordhorst CH, Thygeson P: Infection of rhesus and cynomolgus monkeys with egg-grown viruses of trachoma and inclusion conjunctivitis. Ann NY Acad Sci 98:167, 1962

Dawson CR, Schachter J: TRIC agent infections of the eye and genital tract. Am J Ophthalmol 63:1288, 1967

Dawson CR, Schachter J, Ostler H et al: Inclusion conjunctivitis and Reiter's syndrome in a married couple. Arch Ophthalmol 83:300, 1970

Dawson CR, Thygeson P, Wood R et al: Keratitis and other complications in volunteers infected with inclusion conjunctivitis agent. Rev Int Trach 44:7, 1967

Dunlop EMC, Vaughan-Jackson JD et al: Chlamidiae in non-specific urethritis. Br J Vener Dis 48:425, 1972

Furness G, Graham D, Reeve P, Collier LH: The growth of trachoma and inclusion blennorrhea viruses in cell culture. Rev Int Trach 4:574, 1960a

Furness G, Graham DM, Reeve P: The titration of trachoma and inclusion blennorrhoea viruses in cell cultures. J Gen Microbiol 23:613, 1960b

Gordon FB, Quan AL, Trimmer RW: Morphological observation on trachoma virus in cell culture. Science 131:733, 1960

Halberstädter L, Prowazek S: Ueber Chlamydozoen befunde bei Blennorrhoe neonatorum non gonorrhoica. Berl Klin Wochenschr 46:1839, 1909

Hanna L, Jawetz E, Briones O, et al: Antibodies to TRIC agents in matched human tears and sera. J Immunol 110:1464, 1973

Hanna L, Jawetz E, Thygeson P, Dawson C: Trachoma viruses isolated in United States. I. Growth in embryonated eggs. Proc Soc Exp Biol Med 104: 142, 1960a

Hanna L, Zichosch J, Jawetz E, Vaughan DG Jr, Thygeson P: Virus isolated from inclusion conjunctivitis of newborn (inclusion blennorrhea). Science 132:1660, 1960b

Jawetz E: Seasonal insusceptibility of embryonated eggs to viruses of trachoma and inclusion conjunctivitis. Ann NY Acad Sci 98:31, 1962

Jawetz E, Melnick J, Adelberg E: Review of Medical Microbiology, 4th ed. Los Altos, Cal, Lange Medical Publications, 1960, p 353

Jones BR: Infection by TRIC agents and other members of the Bedsonia group, with a note on Reiter's disease. Trans Ophthalmol Soc UK 86:291, 1966

Jones BR: Trachoma and allied infections. Trans Ophthalmol Soc UK 81:367, 1961

Jones BR, Collier LH: Inoculation of man with inclusion blennorrhea virus. Ann NY Acad Sci 98:212, 1962

Jones BR, Collier LH, Smith CH: Isolation of virus from inclusion blennorrhea. Lancet 1:902, 1959

Julianelle L: A relation of inclusion blennorrhea to swimming-bath conjunctivitis as determined by an accidental transmission. Proc Soc Exp Biol Med 36:617, 1937

Lindner K: Infektions versuche von Trachom mit Paratrachom des Neugeborenen (Einschlussblennorrhoe). Arch Ophthalmol 133:479, 1935

McComb DE, Nichols RL: Antibody type specificity to trachoma in eye secretions of Saudi Arabian children. Infect Immunol 2:65, 1970

Meyer KF: The host spectrum of psittacosis lymphogranuloma venereum. Am J Ophthalmol 63:1225, 1967

Mitsui Y, Suzuki A: Electron microscopy of trachoma virus in section. Arch Ophthalmol 56:429, 1956

Mohsenine H, Darougar S: The provocative effect of cortisone on trachoma. Rev Int Trac 34:336, 1957

Portney GL, Portney SB: Five year perspective on trachoma in the San Xavier Papago Indian. Arch Ophthalmol 92:211, 1974

Schachter JA: Bedsonia isolated from a patient with clinical lymphogranuloma venereum. Am J Ophthalmol 63:1049, 1967

Schachter J, Arnstein P, Dawson C, et al: Human follicular conjunctivitis caused by infection with psittacosis agent. Proc Soc Exp Biol Med 127:292, 1968

Schachter J, Dawson C, Balas S, et al: Evaluation of laboratory methods for detecting acute TRIC agent infection. Am J Ophthalmol 70:375, 1970

Scott JG, Kerrich J: Live trachoma vaccine and topical therapy. Br J Ophthalmol 55:189, 1971

Snyder JC, Bell SD Jr, Murray ES: Attempt to immunize a volunteer (with formalin-inactivated virus) against experimental trachoma induced by Saudi Arabian strain. Ann NY Acad Sci 98:368, 1962

T'ang FF, Chang HL, Huang YT, Wang KC: Studies on the etiology of trachoma, with special reference to isolation of the virus in chick embryo. Chin Med J 75:429, 1957

Thygeson P: Historic review of oculogenital disease. Am J Ophthalmol 71:975, 1971

Thygeson P: The limbus and cornea in experimental and natural human trachoma and inclusion conjunctivitis. Ann NY Acad Sci 98:201, 1962

Thygeson P: The matrix of the epithelial cell inclusion of trachoma. Am J Pathol 14:455, 1938

Thygeson P: The etiology of inclusion blennorrhea. Am J Ophthalmol 17:1019, 1934

Thygeson P, Crocker TT: Observations on experimental trachoma and inclusion conjunctivitis. Am J Ophthalmol 42:76, 1956

Thygeson P, Dawson CR: Trachoma and follicular conjunctivitis in children. Arch Ophthalmol 75:3, 1966

Thygeson P, Hanna L, Dawson C, Zichosch J, Jawetz E: Inoculation of human volunteer with egg-grown inclusion conjunctivitis virus. Am J Ophthalmol 53:786, 1962

Thygeson P, Proctor FI, Richards P: The etiologic significance of the elementary body in trachoma. Am J Ophthalmol 18:811, 1935

Vastine DW, Dawson C, Hoshiwara I, et al: A comparison of media from cases of seasonal conjunctivitis associated with severe endemic trachoma. Appl Microbiol 28:688, 1974

Wang SP, Grayston JT: Human serology in chlamidia trachomatis infection with microimmunofluorescence. J Infec Dis 130:388, 1974

Wang SP, Grayston JT: Pannus with experimental trachoma and inclusion conjunctivitis agent infection of Taiwan monkeys. Am J Ophthalmol 63:1133, 1967

Woolridge RL, Grayston JT: Further studies with a complement-fixation test for trachoma. Ann NY Acad Sci 98:314, 1962

3

Viruses

Viruses cause a great number of infectious diseases of man, animals, and plants. Although we will deal only with agents causing ocular diseases, certain general principles are worthy of mention.

Viruses have been known for many years, but cultivation proved difficult until 1931. In that year, Goodpasture and Woodruff developed the chick embryo technique of viral cultivation, and since then numerous viruses have been isolated. To date, more than 100 viruses are known pathogens for man.

Viruses are particles of matter, primitive yet complicated, living but unique in their mode of replication. Incapable of creating and metabolizing, they must live within cells. Hence, viral diseases are cellular diseases. The study of the virus is intimately related to cellular biochemistry. As Dr. Wendell Stanley has said,

> Viruses, cancer, genes, and life are tied together. . . . Viruses can act as genes, viruses can cause cancer, and viruses are structures at the twilight zone of life partaking both of living and molecular properties.

Besides their individual characteristics, viruses have many common biologic properties. Most viruses may show virulence, mutation, multiplication, host range, specificity, genetic properties, and adaptation to environment. Many, except larger viruses and possibly herpes, are resistant to antibiotics and chemical therapeutic agents.

Chemical Structure of Viruses. In their simplest form, viruses consist of a nucleic acid core surrounded by a protein coat. The nucleic acid, in the form of either DNA or RNA, apparently acts as a template for further viral generation or multiplication. Plant viruses are considered to be among the simplest structures, containing only RNA, while animal viruses have DNA or RNA. Most of the known bacterial viruses (bacteriophages) contain DNA, but some recently studied have RNA. Of the animal viruses, rabbit papilloma virus has the simplest chemical structure and resembles plant viruses.

Viruses containing DNA include (1) the poxvirus group—smallpox, vaccinia, (2) herpesvirus group, (3) adenovirus group, (4) papovavirus group (tumorogenic), and (5) parvovirus and others.

Viruses containing RNA include (1) arbovirus group, (2) orthomyxovirus (isolated from an upper respiratory tract infection, influenza), (3) paramyxovirus group (rubella, measles, and mumps viruses), (4) picornavirus, including enterovirus and others. RNA performs several functions, among which is to act as a messenger for the synthesis of the structure protein.

The larger viruses appear more complicated, and in addition to nucleic acid and proteins, they contain lipids and polysaccharides.

Purification and crystallization of some viruses is a great accomplishment. There are many important methods of purification: precipitation, ultracentrifugation, or column chromatography. The old method of filtrability is of no value, since some bacteria are smaller than large viruses.

Electron microscopy has recently elucidated some formerly invisible structures in viruses. The newly developed negative staining techniques have revealed a great amount of information on their internal structure.

Mutation. The ability to mutate is a characteristic of all forms of life, including viruses. Mutation occurs both in vivo and in tissue culture. A mutation changes the behavior of the virus and may affect its virulence, either enhancing or abating it. For example, the influenza virus differs in virulence every year, and vaccinia virus is a less virulent form than its predecessors. Epidemics may occur when a virus mutates to greater virulence and also changes its antigenic character so that the population at large is susceptible. The range of host animals depends to some degree upon viral mutation. Thus, a virus may, through mutation, adapt to a formerly resistant host.

Knowledge of viral mutation is an important aid to the study of heredity. By experimental mutation through the use of mutagenic agents, viral heredity may be altered.

Interference Phenomenon. When one virus modifies the infected tissue cell in such a way that another virus cannot be an invader, it is called "interference phenomenon." On the other hand, dual viral infections of the same cell may occur (vaccinia and *Herpesvirus simplex*; measles and polioviruses). Isaacs has described an interfering substance, which he named "interferon." He defined it as a normal cell constituent, produced in excess as a defense mechanism in response to viral stimulation, especially if the viral nucleic acid is slightly changed by ultraviolet irradiation. Interferon, produced by one virus, can act against several other viruses. It is a nontoxic protein which can be isolated by conventional methods for protein purification. Isaacs feels also that cells may produce interferon in the absence of the challenging agent. It is now believed that interferon is a protein which stimulates cells to produce another protein called "the translational inhibitory protein" (TIP). This phenomenon differs from specific immunity. It may be possible in the near future to control viral diseases in man, and this is presently the subject of intense study.

Nature and Multiplication of Viruses. Viruses are small structures, being smaller than bacteria but larger than protein molecules, and have no independent metabolism. They therefore are completely dependent upon host cells.

The virus enters a cell as an uninvited guest, demands its nutrition from the cell, and turns it into a factory to produce more viruses. Without a cell, a virus is only an inert particle. Whatever lifelike action can be ascribed to the virus begins as it enters the living cell. Identity remains distinct, and there is no evidence that nucleic acids combine. Rather, the viruses seem to suppress the role of the cell's nucleic acid and redirect the metabolic activities toward viral synthesis. Within the cell, the viral nucleic acid acts as a template for further viral production. The newly formed viral particles emerge from infected cells and in turn affect adjacent cells, and so the cycle repeats until eventually the host cells die or production of antibodies to the viral antigens begins.

Recent work has shown that it is possible to infect cells with isolated purified viral nucleic acid. These results indicate the essential role of the nucleic acid and the secondary protective role of the protein of the viral particle.

Bacteriophage. Bacteria may act as hosts to a special group of viruses, known as "bacteriophages." The phage is highly host-specific. It is probable that all bacteria serve as hosts to one or more phages. The identification of phages is rather complicated and has not yet had much practical use, since phages (except in cholera) have not been therapeutically successful. But this system is ideal for studying the host-parasite relationship and mode of multiplication of viruses (biologic self-reproduction).

Growth of Viruses. Being obligate intracellular parasites, viruses grow only within living (not degenerated or dead) susceptible cells. They have been successfully propagated in various animals as well as in explanted tissues and cells grown in vitro. Tissue cultures and chick embryo membranes, especially chorioallantoic, are the generally used culture media. During their host cells' period of active growth and metabolism, viral growth probably ceases when its required substances are exhausted.

Cultivation of viruses and the tissue culture system made possible the preparation of unlimited amounts of vaccines.

Serologic Properties and Tests. Viruses are strongly antigenic and may demonstrate one or more antigens. The ability of some viruses to stimulate antibody formation and thus create immunity is very significant. Immunity against viral infection may be short- or long-lived.

The serologic tests of agglutination, neutralization, complement fixation, and hemagglutination are used in virology. These tests are sensitive and detect viruses in very dilute solution. Unfortunately, many technical difficulties are encountered. Since viruses grow within the cells, their antigens cannot easily be separated from the involved tissue. The antigenic structure may change (mutate), and the virus can thus behave differently from one outbreak to another. Cross reaction frequently occurs with closely related viruses.

Inclusion Bodies. Inclusion bodies, when present, remain a significant diagnostic aid despite the development of other laboratory methods. Negri bodies of rabies are virtually pathognomonic. Also chickenpox and smallpox, often clinically indistinguishable, may readily be diagnosed on the basis of inclusion bodies, which are cytoplasmic in smallpox and intranuclear in chickenpox.

Morphologically, inclusion bodies represent either an aggregation of viral particles (elementary bodies) or a homogeneous mass of undetermined nature. Elementary bodies represent the infectious unit (eg, vaccinia) which can be used to produce the disease experimentally.

According to their staining properties, inclusion bodies are either eosinophilic or basophilic. A single cell may contain one inclusion body or more, generally surrounded by a clear zone. The bodies may be located in the cytoplasm, within the nucleus, or both. They are usually found in epithelial cells.

The cytoplasmic inclusion bodies, chiefly belonging to the group of large viruses, are better known than those bodies residing within the nucleus. It is believed that the basophilic and eosinophilic cytoplasmic inclusion bodies are viral particles (elementary or initial bodies).

The intranuclear inclusion bodies are found chiefly in the small viral groups, especially the neurotropic viruses. They appear in some viruses as eosinophilic homogeneous masses, and their nature is undetermined. They are not thought of as actual viral particles.

Pathology. The pathology caused by viruses is similar to that of other infectious agents. Nevertheless, there are pathologic as well as clinical characteristics that are pathognomonic for certain viruses. These are primarily because of their intracellular habitat.

The purulent process found in most bacterial infections is not typical for viral diseases. Necrosis and proliferation are more common features of viral pathology. Proliferation is usually produced by slow-growing, mildly toxic viruses (Rous sarcoma, or verruca). Since the skin and mucous membranes are the main portals of entry, their epithelial cells are the first attacked. As a result, skin and mucous membrane eruptions and lesions are typical developments.

In tissues or cells grown in vitro, viral infection induces either proliferative or necrotic reactions (plaque formation), and it is by these reactions that viral diagnosis can be ascertained.

Viral infections call forth a typical monocytic cell response. Monocytes are macrophages that clean up tissue debris. Since the viral process is cytopathogenic, causing necrosis, cellular debris is a constant concomitant feature in viral infections. If a purulent process is present simultaneously with viral pathology, it is indicative of secondary bacterial infection. However, the neutrophilic response can be due to necrotic tissue.

Classification. There is no adequate criterion for the accurate classification of viruses. Classification on a basis of general properties divides viruses into groups without particular reference to individual characteristics.

Immunologic properties are supposed to be the main criterion for classification of viruses. With the present progress of serologic study, identification of individual viruses has gradually developed. There is still much confusion; further study of classification is needed.

In practice, classification by symptomatology and organ involvement is still most important for the clinical diagnosis of viral infections. Some diseases present such typical symptomatology that they can be diagnosed clinically without further identification of the virus. On the basis of symptomatology viral diseases are distinguished as either generalized or localized.

The viruses can be distinguished according to the tissue and organ involved. *Enteroviruses:* polio virus, Coxsackie virus, ECHOvirus. *Upper respiratory tract viruses:* influenza, parainfluenza, adenovirus, and the common cold virus. *Localized viral diseases of the skin and mucous membranes: Herpesvirus simplex* Types 1 and 2, varicella-zoster, cytomegaloviruses, molluscum contagiosum, and warts. *Diseases of the salivary glands:* mumps, cytomegalovirus. *Pox group of viruses:* smallpox (variola), vaccinia, and others.

Localized diseases of the eye: adenoviral conjunctivitis, epidemic keratoconjunctivitis, herpetic keratoconjunctivitis, epidemic hemorrhagic conjunctivitis, Newcastle conjunctivitis, and others.

VARIOLA AND VACCINIA

These viruses are closely related but not identical, clinically or biologically. Their origin is not clear, even today. The cowpox virus was used originally by Jenner in 1796 for vaccination against variola. Long-term laboratory propagation by various methods has altered this virus. It is believed that as a result a new vaccinia virus has developed. However, some vaccinial strains probably are derived from smallpox. Differences among the viruses are minor. They produce similar antigens and hemagglutinins which are practically identical in their reaction with immune sera. The difference is in their ease of growth, host range, and, particularly, their clinical manifestation.

Variola

Variola (smallpox) is a highly contagious viral disease which is usually epidemic or endemic. It is primarily a skin disease, with systemic involvement, and has a high mortality. Since Jennerian vaccination the infection has gradually become milder and has a lower mortality.

Variola is an ancient disease well known in China, Central Africa, and India. In the Middle Ages, as a result of the Crusades, variola was widely disseminated throughout Europe and the Middle East. In Central and South America, it was introduced shortly after Columbus' first voyage. Smallpox is still a serious problem in some Asiatic countries, and infections still occur occasionally in Europe and the Americas. In the United States, several epidemics with a high mortality occurred between 1902 and 1930 (Chapin and Smith). The recurrence of epidemics or the number of sporadic cases may vary with public laws governing vaccination.

Clinical Findings. After an incubation period of 10 to 13 days, the toxemia phase begins, characterized by fever and other general symptoms. A few days later, papular eruptions appear, quickly followed by the vesicular and finally the pustular stage. The lesions are distributed through the entire body but occur chiefly on the extremities and face. The eye frequently is involved. The purpuric and hemorrhagic forms of variola are very toxic and usually have a high mortality. Streptococci or other pyogenic bacteria often complicate the process and cause abscesses and pustules.

Findings in the Eye. Primary variola of the eye is unknown, appearing only secondarily to systemic infection. The lids are often involved in the period of eruption. The lesions run the same course as elsewhere: papular, vesicular, and pustular. Severe abscess or gangrene of the lid may occur, usually in association with a bacterial infection. Variola of the lids may result in permanent scarring and consequent trichiasis and symblepharon (Saxena RC et al). Keratitis and conjunctivitis frequently complicate the lid infection.

A catarrhal purulent conjunctivitis is common. In a very toxic infection, bleeding of the conjunctiva may occur, often with an associated bleeding from the nose or mouth.

Conjunctival pustules are rare. When they occur, they are located typically on the bulbar conjunctiva between the limbus and the inner and outer canthus. They resemble phlyctenules but are accompanied by chemosis and severe pain.

The most serious complication of variola is corneal pustule formation. The process is usually bilateral and is often followed by perforation and sometimes by panophthalmitis. As a result, dense adherent leukoma (Plate 25, Fig. 1) or phthisis bulbi may cause total blindness. Numbers of blind persons with pitted faces and corneal leukoma can be seen in countries where there have been epidemics of smallpox. The inner eye, particularly the uveal tract, is rarely involved. Albinotic spots of the iris as a consequence of variola have been recorded in 50 percent of cases (Duke-Elder).

Laboratory Studies. The host range is virtually restricted to man and monkeys. Animals other than monkeys have only slight susceptibility to the variola virus. As a result, the virus has not been intensively studied. However, growth of the virus on chorioallantoic membrane has been achieved (Buddingh; Lazarus et al). Whitish lesions were produced, smaller than those of vaccinia and with central necrosis. The variola virus is stable and can be propagated from dried specimens even more than one year old. Variola can be confused with varicella, meningococcemia, drug rash, and other skin eruptions. Cultural characteristics and specific antibodies are the most distinctive laboratory methods of differential diagnosis.

Cytoplasmic or intranuclear eosinophilic guarnieri inclusion bodies, or both, are usually found in epithelial cells from the smallpox pustule base. These bodies are large, circular or oval, homogeneous or granular, eosinophilic masses, one or more in number. Before Paschen's study, they were often regarded as protozoan in nature. In 1906 Paschen described elementary bodies, which are now generally recognized as a unit of the virus. These minute bodies are always found in great numbers in the fluid from the variola and vaccinia vesicles. Paschen also concluded that the guarnieri bodies consist of viral elementary bodies. Mononuclear cells, ballooning degeneration of epithelium, and marked necrosis are additional findings. Neutrophils predominate in the pustules (Plate 25, Fig. 4).

The electron microscope can be used for rapid differentiation of variola from chickenpox.

It is believed that viral multiplication occurs twice: first in the cells at the site of the portal of entry or within reticuloendothelial cells. From here the viruses invade the bloodstream and then spread into the skin, where the second multiplication takes place.

Treatment.   There is no specific therapy for variola. Convalescent serum, even in large amounts, has no effect on the infection. Prevention or treatment of bacterial complications by sulfonamides and antibiotics is important.

Vaccinia immunoglobulin (VIG) can prevent or diminish the severity of the disease. It must be given as soon as possible after exposure to infection.

To prevent variola, primary vaccination is given between the ages of four and six months but preferably between 4 and 6 years to avoid serious complications. In some countries where epidemics no longer occur vaccination is no longer considered necessary, but in an endemic area vaccination should be carried out.

When ocular involvement occurs, topical therapy is added to the general treatment of the disease.

Vaccinia

Vaccinia refers to the infections caused by the virus propagated in laboratories for prophylaxis against smallpox. The origin of this virus is obscure. It is presumably cowpox virus, altered by transmission from man to man and to laboratory animals. As a result, a new entity, vaccinia virus, developed.

The main function of the vaccinia virus is to induce immunity against the smallpox virus, to which it is antigenically closely related. This suggests that some vaccinial strains have derived from the smallpox virus.

Clinical Features.   The clinical manifestations of vaccinia occur following vaccination, autovaccination, or contact contamination.

The original vaccination lesion may be complicated by pyogenic organisms, with resultant cellulitis, ulceration, or severe necrosis. The use of dressings on the site of inoculation can create a condition for the growth of tetanus. In the individual who has no ability to produce antibodies to the vaccinia virus, a gangrenous process may develop (Laurance et al).

Systemic reactions, such as urticarial and erythematous rashes, often result from routine vaccinations. The most severe, but fortunately rare, complications are encephalomyelitis and generalized vaccinia.

Vaccinial encephalomyelitis is similar clinically to those of variola and measles. There are several suggestions as to its origin: from the vaccinia virus itself, from allergy, or by activation of another dormant neurotropic virus. Encephalomyelitis is more likely to occur if vaccination is done at a very early age, under 2 or 3 years. Fetal vaccinia infection can develop if the mother has been inoculated within 3 to 24 weeks of gestation.

Generalized vaccinia, sometimes with high mortality, may occur in persons having dermatoses of varied origin, including trauma. This also can develop merely by contact with a vaccinated person (Sommerville et al).

In a case of autovaccination the virus from the lesion of vaccination may spread to other parts of the body, including the eye. Transmission is caused by direct inoculation following scratching or rubbing of the original lesions.

Findings in the Eye.   Vaccinia infections of the eye may occur either by autovaccination or, more frequently, by contact contamination (Rosen). The lids are most likely to become infected and pustules to develop about three days after vaccination. The pustules are usually localized to the skin of the inner angulus of the lower lid (Plate 25, Fig. 3). Occasionally a few coalescent lesions may develop. Severe swelling of the lids, preauricular and submaxillary glands, and other systemic symptoms accompany the process. Stenosis of the lacrimal passage is a rare complication of the vaccinial lesion in the inner angulus of the lower lid.

Ulcerative blepharitis is another type of vaccinial complication. The ulcers are frequently covered by gray, necrotic membranes. Purulent conjunctivitis is commonly associated with the blepharitis.

A purulent conjunctivitis without blepharitis has frequently been observed. An ulcer may occur on the lower conjunctiva. Vaccinial conjunctivitis which developed in the absence of lid lesions has been reported (Groffead and Harrison).

The cornea is seldom directly infected from the original vaccinial lesion. More often, such infection is secondary to infection of the lid and conjunctiva. The keratitis is manifested in three forms: marginal, disciform (Perera) (Plate 25, Fig. 2), or as a corneal pustule. A pustule of the cornea is a serious condition, which may result in perforation of the cornea and possibly blindness. Fortunately, the incidence is rare, and it is usually associated with a corneal abrasion.

Pseudoretinitis pigmentosa with a good prognosis is recorded as an extremely rare complication of vaccination. The eye, particularly the inner part and nerve tissue, may be involved in cases of vaccinial encephalitis.

Laboratory Studies. In contrast to variola, vaccinia virus can successfully infect many animals. Those used most extensively in experiments are rabbits and monkeys. Rabbits in particular are highly susceptible to vaccinia, and they readily develop an acute keratitis after vaccinial inoculation of the scarified cornea. This method can therefore be used for quick diagnosis of vaccinial infection. Numerous vaccinia inclusion bodies are frequently found, which confirm the diagnosis. Vaccinia grows readily on chorioallantoic membrane. The virus may also be cultivated successfully in tissue culture, particularly tissue from rabbit testes or kidney tissues (van Rooyen and Rhodes).

Vaccinia virus has been adapted to grow in almost any type of tissue cells. Dermal and neural vaccinia strains have been recently developed. The effect of neural strains is best studied in monkeys.

Guarnieri variola-vaccinia eosinophilic cytoplasmic inclusion bodies consist of Paschen's elementary bodies. Inclusion bodies in vaccinia are usually cytoplasmic, while in variola they can be intranuclear as well (Plate 25, Fig. 4). The latter are often found in cells at the base of the vesicles, while the cytoplasmic bodies are observed in cells located more superficially in the epithelial layers. These findings are quite specific in vaccinia, having been studied extensively in keratitis of rabbits. They can also be demonstrated in the epithelium of various parts of the body, eg, skin, conjunctiva, sebaceous cysts, meibomian glands, and from the mucous membranes of the nose and throat.

Treatment. There is no specific effective treatment. A child should be cautioned not to rub his eyes. Immune gamma globulin may be of value particularly in generalized vaccinia. For the ophthalmologist, the objective is to prevent the spread of infection from the site of inoculation. Good general hygiene of the skin should be emphasized. The usual treatment by lotion, antibiotics, or other aseptic ointment is recommended.

HERPESVIRUS SIMPLEX

Manifestations of *Herpesvirus simplex* infection are frequent and varied. There are several clinical entities, characterized by vesicular eruptions of the skin and mucous membranes. These variations are due to virulence of the strain, degree of local immunity, and history of previous attack. *Herpesvirus simplex* commonly infects the eye, having a special predilection for the cornea.

In the United States, herpetic keratitis is a troublesome, often chronic disease and is a frequent cause of blindness (Braley). Its incidence and severity appear to be increasing. Thygeson et al (1953) and Kimura et al feel the increasing frequency coincides with recent wars and the antibiotic and steroid eras. It is also associated with an increase in the incidence of venereal diseases (Wilkie et al). There has been a marked increase in genital *H. simplex* and in neonatal infection, varying from mild to fatal (Hagler et al) and from keratoconjunctivitis to necrotizing chorioretinitis in the eye.

As a result of intensive study, a new classification of diseases and strains has developed. There are two distinguishable types: (1) oral and (2) genital *H. simplex* viruses. Unfortunately this classification is not clear yet, particularly concerning sources of infection in association with primary or recurrent types of *H. simplex*.

Clinical Features. *H. simplex* infection is divided clinically into primary herpes and recurrent herpes.

PRIMARY *H. SIMPLEX* INFECTION. Initial or primary herpes infection usually occurs in children aged six months to 5 years and may occur in adolescence; it is rare in adulthood. Infants appear to be born with maternal herpes-specific antibodies which disappear within six months. From then to 24 months, sensitivity to herpes infection is greatest. Gingivostomatitis, vulvovaginitis, Kaposi's eruption (eczema herpeticum), and acute keratoconjunctivitis (Gallardo) are common primary herpes manifestations. These are usually accompanied by systemic involvement, fever, and enlargement of regional glands. The infection can be severe, even fatal. Nevertheless, about 90 percent of primary herpes cases are asymptomatic.

Severe infection may occur in premature infants, and a fatal viremia may result. The mechanism is not known, but possibly there is a low titer of maternal antibodies, a high dose of the virus, or, according to Rake, greater vulnerability of premature cells. The disease may be associated with herpes of the maternal genitalia. Type 2 *H. simplex* (genital) is associated with (1) genital herpes (herpes progenitalis) and (2) neonatal herpes, which develops by contact with herpetic lesions in the birth canal. Type 2 *H. simplex* usually does not produce lesions in extragenital locations in adults. However, it has been reported in adults as the cause of acute blepharoconjunctivitis (Oh et al) and acute keratoconjunctivitis, in which genital transmission was proven by positive culture.

After the first attack in infants, antibodies against *H. simplex* are demonstrated. This was confirmed when Buddingh et al reported the presence of neutralizing antibodies in 90 percent of healthy persons over the age of 15. The finding of specific antibodies is regarded as evidence of previous primary herpes infection. It is also recognized that primary herpes gives rise to a latent infection that may persist throughout life. This may be activated by many unspecific stimuli and becomes recurrent. Latent virus in the cornea is not the only source of recurrent herpetic infection, since the virus has been isolated from saliva and tears (Kaufman et al, 1968).

RECURRENT *H. SIMPLEX* INFECTION.   Common factors appearing to reactivate the latent *H. simplex* are various fevers—pneumonia, malaria, or others—emotional disturbances, physical trauma, such as cold or heat, chemical factors, drugs, such as epinephrine, and others. The exact mechanism of activation is unknown. The evidence of recurrent infection is the presence of specific antibodies in convalescent serum (Andrewes and Carmichael). During the primary attack, antibodies appear about 10 days after onset. The recurrent process is usually localized and without systemic involvement. The commonest clinical entities are herpes febrilis, herpes labialis, herpes genitalis, and herpes of the cornea.

If chronic eczema is present, *H. simplex* infection causes a severe condition called "eczema herpeticum."

Findings in the Eye. *H. simplex* has a primary affinity for the cornea, causing a dendritic keratitis which is pathognomonic.

In primary infection, dendritic keratitis occurs rarely, and seldom before six months of age. However, it has been recognized in premature infants. In infancy and childhood, the process is usually bilateral and more severe than in adults (Plate 27, Fig. 1). It is accompanied by systemic manifestations, enlargement of regional nodes, or occasionally by central nervous system involvement.

Superficial (epithelialis) punctate or diffuse keratitis has also been considered a primary manifestation of *H. simplex* infection. The same clinical picture can be found in other conditions, particularly epidemic keratoconjunctivitis. Therefore, laboratory diagnosis is necessary. However, loss of corneal sensitivity may distinguish herpetic keratitis from epidemic keratoconjunctivitis.

An acute follicular conjunctivitis is usually found with primary herpetic keratitis in children, but adult primary herpetic keratitis is often associated with an acute ulcerative blepharitis. It was found recently that primary *H. simplex* infection may occur in adolescents and young adults not as rarely as was believed.

In recurrent infection, dendritic keratitis is the commonest ocular sign. This condition occurs unilaterally, predominantly in adult males (Plate 27, Fig. 2). Regional lymph nodes are uninvolved, and there is no systemic symptomatology. However, keratoconjunctivitis has been reported with severe systemic involvement in young adults 29 to 30 years of age (Howard). The keratitis evolves as a superficial punctate type with erosions. Within 24 hours a small dendritic ulcer may develop. Vesicles in groups or rows may appear prior to ulceration, but they rupture promptly and often escape detection. The branches of the dendritic figure have knobby extremities; iris usually involved.

The herpetic process is usually chronic and recurrent and not very clear. A possible additional explanation appears to have been neglected. The virus can be neurotropic and usually affects the central cornea, which is richest in nerve branches. As a result, the keratitis is primarily neurotrophic, as evidenced by loss of sensitivity. It is known that neurotrophic keratitis of any origin presents a problem of recurrence. Dendritic keratitis, even mild, is usually followed by scarring (Plate 27, Fig. 7). However, it may be complicated by secondary bacterial or fungal infection, which may result from steroid therapy. Steroid therapy, particularly in the early stages of a herpetic keratitis, is quite dangerous. Thygeson pointed out that hypopyon keratitis may present a diagnostic problem if a preceding dendritic keratitis has not been observed. Total corneal anesthesia and an indolent process are clues to prior herpes infection.

Besides dendritic keratitis there is a variety of herpetic keratitides, both superficial and interstitial (Thygeson et al, 1956; Metcalf et al). Among the superficial types (Ormsby) are punctate, erosions, marginal, striatum, stellatum, band-shaped, and filamentous. The filamentous form develops perhaps as a result of prolonged edema or too frequent cauterization. The function of the lacrimal glands is usually normal. The herpetic keratitides are often confused with similar conditions of other etiology. Braley (1957) pointed out that superficial punctate keratitis may often be mistaken for epidemic keratoconjunctivitis. Among the deep herpetic keratitides, disciform is most frequent (Plate 27, Fig. 6). Thygeson and Kimura regard disciform keratitis as principally caused by *H. simplex* and only rarely caused by vaccinia, mumps, or varicella-zoster. Benign and severe disciform types of herpetic keratitis occur. In the latter, necrosis and perforation are seen. The increasing number of severe cases recently reported may follow steroid therapy. Several authors indicate that disciform keratitis may be associated with hypersensitivity or frequent use of iodine cauterization.

Herpetic infections of the eye are distinguished by Hogan et al as follows: *Superficial:* (1) dendritic keratitis with or without stromal involvement and (2) geographic epithelial keratitis (late superficial). *Deep keratitis:* stromal without ulceration (disciform) or with ulceration (perforated or nonperforated). *Uveitis:* with or without keratitis both ulcerated and nonulcerated.

The stromal lesion might be caused either by the interaction of viral antibodies, both humoral and cellular, or by the direct consequence of viral multiplication (Tanaka, Kimura), causing cell death and the release of toxic products. The way in which the virus enters is not understood.

It has been shown that cell-mediated allergy plays a significant role in the pathology of herpetic infection.

Herpetic conjunctivitis, common in children, is rarely seen in adults. It is either a follicular (Plate 28, Fig. 2) or, less frequently, a membranous type, and neither is distinguishable from similar manifestations of other origin. Prior or simultaneous appearance of vesicular skin eruptions is diagnostically important. Vesicles are occasionally seen on the palpebral conjunctiva. These promptly break down, leaving superficial ulcers.

Acute herpetic blepharitis may be found in adults (Plate 28, Fig. 3), being characterized by formation of vesicles along the cilial lines. The vesicles break down and ulcerate. The ulcers are covered by glistening grayish membranes, which have a tendency to spread over the palpebral conjunctiva. The lid margins become edematous and a concurrent dermatitis of the upper lid is often present. Some of our cases also showed marked enlargement of the preauricular glands (oculoglandular Parinaud's syndrome).

Recurrent indolent herpetic iritis and iridocyclitis of a hemorrhagic type are recorded. They often result in secondary glaucoma. These are usually preceded by severe disciform keratitis.

A case of recurrent sympathetic ophthalmia due to *H. simplex* has been described (Cavara et al).

New clinical herpetic diseases have been reported: congenital cataract (Cibis and Burde), bilateral chorioretinitis followed by encephalitis in which Type 2 *H. simplex* was isolated (Cogan et al), congenital keratoconjunctivitis of Type 1 probably acquired in utero, since the mother had no genital herpes (Hutchison et al).

There is a report of recurrent herpetic keratitis associated with the menstrual cycle (Deutsch), ceasing after administration of ovarian hormone. *H. simplex* may cause endothelial vesicles (Kiffney).

METAHERPES. The term "metaherpes" refers to the keratitis which develops on the site of a healed dendritic keratitis. This appears in various forms, mainly as superficial round or oval ulcers, often with scalloped borders, but not in a dendritic form. Superficial infiltrates or a deep interstitial process may be seen. Metaherpes develops slowly, and contrary to the condition in dendritic keratitis, epithelial cells are more firmly fixed. The process does not heal readily, and its etiology is unknown. In some cases it can be an allergic manifestation. Since metaherpes occurs in the area of anesthesia, the keratitis is possibly neuroparalytic. Hogan regards the name "metaherpes" as confusing and would prefer to designate the process "chronic postherpetic corneal ulceration."

Current Developments. Current development in laboratory diagnosis is given in an excellent review by Howard and Kaufman.

H. simplex is dermotropic, but virulent strains may become neurotropic. *H. simplex* has a wide range of susceptible hosts. It grows readily on the chorioallantoic membrane of 10- to 13-day old embryonated eggs (Scott et al), producing plaques containing Lipschütz inclusion bodies. It can also be propagated in tissue culture (Doane et al), chick embryo or rabbit kidney tissue being considered best. Hanna et al have shown the advantage of HeLa cell culture in detecting both *H. simplex* and adenovirus.

Rabbit cornea has been widely used experimentally because of its marked susceptibility to *H. simplex.* Viral inoculation of the scarified cornea causes severe keratitis within 24 hours. Propagation of the virus can be achieved by passages. Rabbits are now used less because of the advantages of new techniques, such as tissue culture techniques.

The fact that *H. simplex* has been isolated from healthy carriers must be considered in establishing its etiologic role.

The method of collecting specimens is important. Swabbed or scraped material must be collected in the acute state. Culture medium 199 is the most suitable for preserving specimens. This can serve as inoculum for embryonated eggs, animals, and tissue culture. The use of saline is not recommended, since it may inhibit the growth of the virus. The specimen should be studied as early as possible, but if necessary it can be stored for a short time in the freezer compartment of the refrigerator.

Cytologic study is based on scrapings and sections. For the scrapings, Giemsa stain is commonly used. The inclusion bodies are better demonstrated by Papanicolaou's (PAP) stain. One finds homogeneous intranuclear eosinophilic masses described by Lipschütz as *H. simplex* inclusion bodies. These are now regarded as the end stage of a two-stage viral development. In the first stage, the inclusion bodies appear as a basophilic Feulgen-positive substance (DNA) consisting of viral particles. In the second stage, these particles gradually disappear and are replaced by a nonviral Feulgen-negative eosinophilic mass (Lipschütz bodies), thought to be a product of cellular degeneration caused by the virus. It has also been referred to as a "nuclear scar."

Lipschütz bodies are easily demonstrated experimentally, but rarely, and usually in an early stage in human herpes infection. Giant cells containing 2 to 15 or more nuclei are regarded as significant for *H. simplex* (Plate 27, Figs. 4, 5). Consistent demonstration of these cells in corneal, conjunctival, or skin scrapings may justify the diagnosis. A special method for staining the scrapings is described by Lennette and van Allen. Ballooning degeneration of epithelial cells as a result of fluid collection may be a diagnostic aid. Polynuclear cells are often found in association with secondary bacterial infection. Cytologic examination has some value, especially in association with other diagnostic data (Plate 27, Fig. 3).

Serologic Study. Type 1 (oral) and Type 2 (genital) are distinguishable serologically and epidemiologically by their growth requirements and sensitivity to heat (Type 2 being the more sensitive). Antibodies to Type 1 are most commonly found in adults. Antibodies to Type 2 appear in adolescence. It was found, in experimental work on rabbits, that Type 1 causes superficial keratitis of early onset with rapid healing without scarring. Type 2 causes much more severe keratitis of longer duration with stromal involvement, pannus, and scarring (Oh and Stevens; Stevens and Oh).

Coons et al reported fluorescenin-labeled antibodies. The fluorescein antibody technique has the highest sensitivity and may be more valuable than viral isolation, which is very time-consuming. Viral particles have been demonstrated by fluorescence in electron microscopic investigation in the corneal stroma (Font; Tanaka and Kimura).

The question of immunity is in doubt, as recurrent *H. simplex* infection is very frequent. However, it has been demonstrated that recurrent lesions do not commonly appear on the same site, and if they do occur, the infection is shorter and milder. Also, a number of specific antibodies have been found in convalescent sera. There are many theories on recurrence of herpes: (1) the antibody titer is probably low, (2) antibodies are not completely specific, (3) some viruses have a very high virulence, (4) immunity is confined to the area of the healed lesions. At present no satisfactory explanation is available.

It is believed that in the herpetic diseases, host sensitivity plays a more active role than do the viruses themselves. The first report of pathologic study of herpetic retinopathy (Cogan et al) shows that the process is immunologic rather than a direct infection by the virus.

Treatment. Numerous remedies have been advocated for treatment of dendritic keratitis. The reader is referred to a comprehensive discussion of older methods of the treatment by Thomas. Iodine therapy was a popular method. Its purpose is to destroy the epithelial cells harboring the viruses. Therefore the corneal epithelial cells of the involved and adjacent areas, sometimes of the entire cornea, have to be removed. The epithelial cells are loosely connected with the cornea and therefore easily denuded. First, anesthetize the cornea; then use a fine applicator wetted with tincture of iodine. Cauterization must be done thoroughly to obtain a good result. After cauterization, repeated instillation of 4 percent cocaine hydrochloride is recommended by Thomas. This precipitates iodides, with a resultant dark brown color of the area. Epithelial cells are quickly regenerated, and healing usually follows without scarrring. Atropine drops and light bandaging complete the procedure. At present this method is not used by a majority of ophthalmologists.

Surgical treatments, such as lamellar grafting (Hogan et al; Peister et al), and penetrating keratoplasty are mostly not successful.

Gamma globulin, administered topically and parenterally, has not been particularly useful. Antibiotics are used chiefly for secondary bacterial infections, since they have no recognized specific effect on any type of *H. simplex*. However, very encouraging results have been recorded with IDU (5-iodo-2'-deoxyuridine) (Kaufman et al, 1962). IDU and corticosteroid therapy of *H. simplex* infections has become widely used. Both have positive and negative results, and their application has to be chosen with proper care.

IDU has beneficial effects in the early stage of herpetic keratitis, being more successful against Type 1. It does not prevent recurrence and inhibits cell regeneration, prolonging healing of the corneal ulcer (Hughes). Allergy to IDU has been observed to take the form of chronic follicular conjunctivitis, with swollen lids and obstruction of the punctum lacrimale. Recurrence of keratitis may follow IDU therapy (Carroll et al). The application of adenine-arabinoside (ARA-A) may be useful in case of resistance to IDU. It has the advantages over IDU of providing better tissue penetration and of showing a lack of toxicity (Langston et al; Kaufman et al, l962).

Steroids may increase viral replication, enhance invasion by the virus, increase complication by bacterial and fungal infection, and inhibit interferon production. They are contraindicated in dendritic keratitis and should be used carefully only in combination with IDU. They are most beneficial in deep keratitis without ulceration.

The virus is relatively resistant to interferon (Kaufman et al, 1969). There is no evidence that cryotherapy is superior to any other debridement method.

The effects of these mentioned treatments are only partial, and knowledge of better methods is urgently needed.

Thygeson recommends that at the early onset of superficial keratitis the use of mydriatics and patching of the eye rather than more drastic treatment can be very effective.

VARICELLA-ZOSTER GROUP

Cultural and serologic investigation led Weller in 1953 to the conclusion that the zoster and varicella viruses are identical. It has been shown that inoculation of zoster vesicle fluid into infants, varicellalike diseases may develop, as may happen after contact with patients having herpes zoster. This has not happened in children convalescing from varicella. However, adults frequently initiate epidemics of varicella. The relationship between the viruses of varicella and zoster is similar to that of *H. simplex* in its primary and recurrent forms. Varicella (chickenpox) is a primary manifestation in children. Then, the virus becomes latent, being localized within nerve cells. Various stimulating factors, such as breast cancer, leukemia, intramuscular injections, trauma, or others, can cause the latent viruses to be manifested as zoster (shingles). In patients with zoster, it is also advisable to check for leukemia or breast cancer (Blodi, Kielar et al).

Clinical Features (Scheie H).   Zoster is characterized by skin or mucous membrane vesicular lesions distributed along one or more groups of sensory nerves. Simultaneously, the dorsal roots of the trunk or dorsal ganglia are involved. Zoster is most frequently manifested on the neck, shoulders, and arms, the process usually being unilateral. The incubation period is not fully established. Severe pain is typical at the onset of the condition, then vesicles appear. They become ulcerated and covered by crusts, and scarring may ensue (Bonzas). Early in the disease the lymph nodes of the involved area are enlarged. In older subjects, persistent neuralgia is usual in convalescence.

Clinical features of varicella are subjects for the pediatrician and therefore will not be discussed here. Ocular involvements are rare, but vesicles are nearly always present on the lid as part of the general skin eruption. Temporary blindness may be associated with an encephalitis, which is an occasional complication of varicella. It must be emphasized that steroid therapy should be avoided. Fatal results have been reported, especially when the varicella was complicated by pneumonia (Haggerty and Eley).

Findings in the Eye.   Zoster ophthalmicus is usually an acute unilateral and severe process characterized by vesicular eruptions along the ophthalmic branches of the trigeminus nerve (Plate 26, Fig. 1). Frequently the gasserian ganglion is inflamed with ocular involvement. The lids and cornea are most often involved, and the conjunctiva is rarely affected. The vesicles occur at the inner half of the lid if the supratrochlear branch is involved. Follicles and pustules may appear on the superior tarsal conjunctiva, and bulbar lesions appear at the limbus. Episcleritis or scleritis may develop at the onset or in the later stages, particularly after the withdrawal of steroid therapy. This has a tendency to be chronic (Marsh). If the nasociliar branch is attacked, keratitis may result. This is manifested mainly as subepithelial, discrete infiltrates or in the form of a discus nummularis in the epithelium, consisting of punctate dots. Simultaniously, vesicles in rows or groups are occasionally seen. They rupture rapidly, forming superficial ulcers. Neuroparalytic ulcerative keratitis may develop in more severe cases. These ulcers may be easily complicated by secondary bacterial infection, resulting in hypopyon keratitis. Interstitial disciform keratitis, although rare, appears mainly as a severe process, accompanied by Descemet's folds (Plate 26, Fig. 2). It develops within one or more weeks after the onset of zoster and is probably of allergenic origin. Disciform keratitis is frequently complicated by iridocyclitis (Klein and Farkas) and glaucoma. In any of these keratitides, scarring and a marked decrease of sensitivity are typical. Rarely, central or peripheral keratitis with immune rings occurs and tends to become chronic.

The cornea is involved in about 35 percent of cases. Three major courses of keratitis may occur: acute, chronic, and relapsing.

Dendritic keratitis, usually considered as pathognomonic for *H. simplex* infection, is a new development in zoster (Plate 26, Fig. 3) from which zoster virus was isolated (Pavan-Langston and McCulley), but it is still difficult to diagnose, since *H. simplex* dendritic keratitis can be superimposed on zoster keratitis, often provoked by steroid treatment. Some distinctive characteristics may be helpful (Piebanga and Laibson): in zoster small, single or multiple dendritic ulcers usually appear at the limbus (Marsh), whereas in *H. simplex* infection they appear in the center. Zoster ulcers show dull, irregular fluorescent staining, and *H. simplex* ulcers are brightly fluorescent. In zoster, corneal edema is diffuse; in *H. simplex* infection, it is local. Tear films in zoster make dry spots on the corneal epithelium in spite of a normal Shirmer test. Steroid treatment does not reactivate the zoster keratitis and does not respond to IDU. Therefore, the differential diagnosis of *H. simplex* and zoster dendritic keratitis is important in determining treatment.

Relapsing keratitis may occur at different periods after the onset from weeks to several years. It occurs as an indolent ulcer in the palpebral space. The entire cornea can be involved, and sensitivity can be totally lost (Marsh). Often relapses are associated with the withdrawal of steroid treatment.

Pemberton has reported another rare involvement—an obstruction of the central artery and vein, detachment of the retina, local choroiditis, internal ophthalmoplegia, and optic nerve atrophy.

The diagnosis of ocular zoster is often determined by the presence of typical skin manifestations.

Involvement of the eye in chickenpox is rare (Rogers). A mild conjunctivitis or vesicular keratitis may occur. These are usually associated with lid eruptions and disappear rapidly (Plate 26, Fig. 5). When varicella-zoster viral diseases are complicated by encephalitis, ocular motor paralyses are frequent. The optic nerve is rarely affected.

Laboratory Studies. The virus has not been found to produce disease in any species other than man. It was first transmitted to volunteers (children) by Steiner in 1875. Weller, 1953, first grew viruses of varicella and zoster in the cell culture of human embryonic tissue. He found that both viruses produced had the same type of cytopathogenic effect. Goodpasture and Anderson accomplished growth of the zoster virus in skin grafted onto the chorioallantois of chick embryos. It is not propogated in laboratory animals. Fluorescent antibody technique gave evidence of the mutual antibody relationship of the varicella and zoster viruses.

Intranuclear Lipschütz inclusion bodies, similar to those of *H. simplex* are found. Their relationship to viral multiplication is not sufficiently clear, as similar inclusion bodies have appeared in some non-viral conditions. The development of inclusion bodies is the same as in *H. simplex* (p. 203). Ballooning cell degeneration, giant multinucleated cells, and many polymorphonuclear cells are also found (Plate 26, Fig. 4).

Rapid differentiation between the zoster virus and *H. simplex* is made by examination of vesicle fluid with the electron microscope for the presence of viral particles and by isolation of the virus. The use of the immunofluorescent technique for specific antibodies may be helpful (Hayashi et al; Weller, 1954). It can demonstrate EgM and EgG in varicella and EgG in zoster. The histopathology of zoster ophthalmicus has been reported.

Immunity. Both varicella and zoster usually produce a lasting immunity. Nevertheless, the varicella virus under certain conditions may relapse.

Treatment. Ocular zoster does not respond to IDU. Steroid therapy can be used in any kind of keratitis, but it can sometimes activate latent *H. simplex*. To avoid a relapse after steroid withdrawal, treatment should be continued for at least six months after healing. Zoster iritis does not usually respond to steroids.

Zoster immunoglobulins (ZIG) can be used to prevent or modify the illness in children with immunologic dysfunction or in children who are exposed to varicella while under antimetabolite or steroid therapy.

The eruptions of zoster and varicella require care in the prevention of secondary bacterial infection. If such infection has already developed, sulfonamides and the proper antibiotics are used. Personal hygiene, especially of the skin, is an important measure. Sedative ointments are indicated in severe pain. Section of the sensory root may be required if chronic neuralgia develops.

ADENOVIRUS GROUP

Adenoviruses are medically important viruses, having been isolated by tissue culture techniques. The first isolation was reported by Rowe and his co-workers in 1953. The agents, found in fragments of surgically removed human adenoids, were initially called "adenoid degeneration viruses." Almost simultaneously, Hilleman and Werner, also by tissue culture technique, isolated a virus from Army recruits having acute respiratory disease (ARD). In the same year Huebner et al studied a clinical entity for which they suggested the name "adeno-pharyngeal-conjunctivitis" (APC). The name "adenovirus," proposed by Enders et al, has been generally accepted since 1956.

Adenoviral infection is worldwide, causing mainly respiratory tract and eye diseases—acute respiratory diseases (ARD) and pharyngoconjunctival fever (PCF). ARD and PCF often occur in epidemic form and have some clinical symptoms in common. These include fever and lymphadenopathy.

Findings in the Eye.   Following the isolation of adenoviruses, intensive studies of eye involvements were made, particularly in the United States (Jawetz, Thygeson, Kimura, et al) and in Japan (Mitsui, Tanaka, et al). The most common adenoviral infection of children is PCF. This is characterized by the triad pharyngitis, conjunctivitis, and fever. The incubation period is from 2 to 10 days. Mild pharyngitis is accompanied by adenopathy, usually submaxillary. It is often associated with high fever, even to 104 F. The child may have coryza, gastrointestinal disturbances, or meningismus.

The conjunctivitis is follicular (Plate 28, Fig. 4) often unilateral, and usually involves the lower fornix. It lasts about three weeks. The other eye may become involved, usually not so severely, two to five days after onset of the condition. A superficial transitory corneal opacity may be present. Serologic type 3 is the principal cause of PCF.

Epidemics of PCF usually occur during the summer, infecting children 4 to 9 years old. Swimming pools may be a source of infection.

The PCF triad in epidemic form is virtually pathognomonic for adenoviral infection, since the clinical picture is more constant and characteristic in epidemics. More difficult to diagnose are the sporadic cases of PCF, and without laboratory confirmation the diagnosis is only tentative. Sporadic cases of PCF have been studied by Kimura et al. These have mainly involved adults, and in a less severe form than occurs in children. Type 3 adenovirus was isolated from PCF in about half of the cases studied, and types 2 and 6 were occasionally found.

Adenovirus can cause follicular conjunctivitis without systemic symptoms or sore throat, usually occurring in winter, either sporadically or in small epidemics. The preauricular nodes (not maxillary, as in PCF) are enlarged and tender. The infection may occur in epidemic form, the source usually being swimming pools. We have seen several otherwise asymptomatic patients with follicular conjunctivitis in which adenovirus type 3 was isolated. Without isolation of the virus, these cases represent a diagnostic problem, since they are easily confused with herpetic and other follicular conjunctivitides. Important points of differentiation are skin eruptions or acute blepharitis in herpetic infections.

Epidemic keratoconjunctivitis (EKC), another classical triad, has recently been shown to be caused by an adenovirus. The first strain of adenovirus type 8 was isolated from epidemic keratoconjunctivitis by Jawetz et al (1955). A number of epidemics had already established EKC as a clinical entity. Since these epidemics occurred among shipyard employees, the triad was called the "shipyard disease." Later observations showed that these endemics or epidemics can affect many other persons. Instrument transmission, especially by tonometer, must be avoided.

Classically, a follicular conjunctivitis in the lower fornix initiates the process. Edema of the semilunar fold and caruncula, chemosis, petechiae, and ecchymosis may develop. Systemic involvement is usually lacking.

Pseudomembrane can be a striking manifestation in acute epidemic keratoconjunctivitis (Laibson and Green). A new type of very contagious, acute hemorrhagic keratoconjunctivitis has been reported (Jones, Laibson et al, 1968, Green et al). A severe epidemic uveitis was first observed. Secondary bacterial infection is very common, particularly staphylococcal, which can confuse diagnosis.

The keratitis, which follows 7 to 10 days after onset of the conjunctivitis, is characterized by small, round, discrete, grayish subepithelial infiltrates. The keratitis typically localizes in the pupillary area and may last two to eight weeks or even longer. As a rule it clears without sequelae (Plate 28, Fig. 5).

There has been much discussion as to whether the infiltrates are an inflammatory reaction or viral infections. There is some evidence that electron microscopy has revealed adenoviral particles in a corneal lesion. It was found by Dawson, Hanna and Togni that in southeast Asia presistent corneal erosion similar to recurrent epithelial erosion occurred.

The triad is considered pathognomonic for diagnosis. However, Japanese observers have described a form of EKC in infants which has atypical manifestations (Mitsui and Jawetz; Tanaka). These include a membranous type of conjunctivitis accompanied by systemic symptoms. Most interesting and surprising is the fact that the cornea was not involved. Type 8 adenovirus was, however, isolated. These observers believed the epidemic resulted from swimming pool transmission.

The term EKC has been confused further because diagnosis is often based only on the typical subepithelial, punctate, central keratitis (without conjunctivitis). In such cases, therefore, the term "subepithelial adenoviral keratitis" would be more appropriate. Then this picture could be regarded as pathognomonic in analogy with herpetic dendritic keratitis.

Laboratory Studies. Most attempts to produce adenoviral infections in laboratory animals have failed. Man appears to be the only host for most adenoviruses. Transmission to volunteers has often been positive (Ward et al), especially in the case of conjunctivitis. Mitsui et al produced keratitis in volunteers by inoculation of type 8 isolated from EKC.

Cultivation of adenoviruses has been successful in monkey kidney tissue and rabbit trachea epithelial cells. In tissue culture of human cells, the virus produces characteristic cytopathic changes more rapidly than in fibroblasts, also in HeLa cells. Inclusion bodies have been found in positive tissue culture. They are eosinophilic and are initially Feulgen-negative, later becoming basophilic Feulgen-positive. The electron microscope shows viral particles in crystalline arrangement.

Adenoviral serologic characteristics have been studied intensively, and as a result, at least 31 serologic types are known that share many serologic and biologic properties. Hence, similar diseases and epidemics are produced by different antigenic types (Enders et al; Golden et al). It is also true that in an epidemic more than one serologic type may be present. The neutralizing antibodies are specific to certain types of the virus.

Most of the adenoviral isolations have been from adenoids and tonsils, which often harbor several serologic types. Their causative role in adenoid hypertrophy has not been proven. Possibly this adenoid tissue serves as a reservoir for latent adenoviruses.

Although there is no constant relationship between the serologic type of virus and the induced disease, one usually finds a predominant type in the epidemic, endemic, or sporadic cases. Types 3 and 7 are epidemic strains in persons of all ages. Types 1 and 2 are endemic strains which are highly contagious (Rose). They infect the majority of children before the age of 2 or 3 years and persist in the adenoids and tonsils. Types 3, 4, 5, 6, and 7 more commonly infect adults. Type 4 is found in acute respiratory diseases of adults, while types 1 and 2 are found in children. In ocular disease, type 3 is a common finding in follicular conjunctivitis and type 8 in EKC (Jawetz et al, 1955). A new type 19 of EKC has been recorded recently (Burn et al; O'Day et al). The variation of serologic types is particularly evident in sporadic cases. In epidemics, the clinical picture and relation to serologic types are usually more constant. Further serologic study is needed for clarification. According to recent data, it would appear that all important serologic types fall into only two major subgroups. The duration of immunity has not been determined.

To determine the specific viral type that caused the infection, neutralization titration must be done with the common types of adenoviruses known to cause infection (Rivers and Horsfall).

Treatment. Antibiotics, convalescent serum, and viral vaccination have no value in treating adenoviral infection. However, antibiotics are indicated in cases of secondary bacterial infection. The treatment is symptomatic. Hot compresses and mydriatics, when indicated, give some relief. There is some controversial data with regard to steroid therapy. It can prolong the process and encourage recurrence of the infection (Laibson et al, 1970).

The principal care must be to increase the patient's general resistance by such factors as sufficient vitamin intake, proper diet, and rest. Any stresses and disturbances of the physical and physiologic balance, including indiscriminate use of new medicines, should be avoided. Variation of seasons, range of age, irritation of mucous membranes, or trauma may be significant contributory factors. Extreme care must be used in cleaning instruments, especially the tonometer (Thygeson).

Vaccination or injection of gamma globulin may be useful in preventing epidemics. Live adenoviral vaccine against types 4 and 7 have been developed and used in military populations. Special epidemiologic circumstances should be decided by an epidemiologist.

MEASLES

Measles, an infectious exanthematous disease usually of childhood, occurs in epidemic form. In debilitated patients and those of low resistance, or when secondary infection occurs (most often *H. influenzae,* staphylococci, or streptococci), the disease can be fatal. The commonest bacterial complications are otitis media, with perforation of the ear drum, and bronchopneumonia. Acute catarrhal conjunctivitis is commonly present. Measles encephalomyelitis is uncommon. It has a high mortality and may cause permanent neurologic damage. Also, measles infection may possibly lower the body's resistance to other infections, such as tuberculosis.

One attack of measles usually confers lifelong immunity. Nevertheless recurrent cases, especially in adults, have been reported.

Clinical Findings.   The incubation period for measles is about 14 days. The prodromal period, the most contagious, is characterized by fever and catarrhal symptoms: conjunctivitis, cough, running nose, and sneezing. Koplik's spots are important for early diagnosis of measles and differentiate measles from rubella (Blank and Rake). They are bluish white, surrounded by scarlet red areolas, and typically localized around the papillae of the parotid duct. However, other mucous membranes, including the conjunctiva, may be involved. These spots represent necrosis of epithelium. The prodromal period lasts from one to five days and is followed by the typical eruption.

Findings in the Eye.   Usually mild, acute, catarrhal, nonpurulent conjunctivitis commonly develops. It is characterized by a severe photophobia, and occasionally, marked edema of the conjunctiva is present. The conjunctivitis is thought to be caused primarily by the virus itself. The process usually subsides when desquamation of the skin begins, but in cases complicated by bacterial infection, severe purulent conjunctivitis may be observed throughout the entire illness. In debilitated children, a severe true membranous conjunctiva may occur. Koplik's spots have been found on the conjunctiva and on the lacrimal caruncula (Duke-Elder). Lid margins may become red and swollen during the conjunctivitis or in the period of eruption. Infectious suppurative inflammation of the meibomian glands sometimes complicates this blepharitis. Gangrene of the lids rarely occurs.

Keratitis is a usual complication. It is mainly a punctate superficial type with multiple epithelial erosions (hence severe photophobia). They can last about two weeks or more after the systemic illness has passed. The keratitis may ulcerate and vascularize. In cases with bacterial contamination or in debilitated children, the keratitis becomes purulent, sometimes followed by panophthalmitis and phthisis bulbi. Metastatic uveitis may occasionally occur.

Laboratory Studies.   The measles virus host range is limited. It has been transmitted to susceptible species of monkeys (Anderson and Goldberger). Cultivation of the virus is difficult, but tissue culture has recently been achieved in monkey and dog kidney tissue. Growth has also been successful on chick embryo chorioallantoic membrane (Rake and Shaffer).

Cytology.   Multinucleated giant cells in the sputum and nasal mucosa during the prodromal period are diagnostically important. In experiments, the giant cells have been found to contain eosinophilic intranuclear inclusion bodies and cytoplasmic eosinophilic masses. Similar inclusion bodies have been described in human specimens (Torres, in Blank and Rake). In measles infection, one finds a monocytic cellular response. The monocytes contain cytoplasmic granules which may be hyalin.

Treatment.   This is usually symptomatic. Warm saline to keep the eye clean is recommended. To relieve the photophobia in cases of keratoconjunctivitis, it is better to keep the patient out of direct light. Antibiotics are necessary in cases of secondary bacterial infection. Gamma globulin together with live vaccine may be effective, particularly in preventing encephalitis. The Enders measles vaccine may eventually eliminate this disease, thus solving the problem of its severe complications.

Prevention of measles by live attenuated virus vaccine represents the most effective control measure.

RUBELLA (GERMAN MEASLES)

There are two types of rubella: (1) postnatal and (2) congenital. Postnatal rubella is an acute febrile disease of children and young adults, characterized by rash and lymphadenopathy. Follicular conjunctivitis or superficial keratitis can be seen, but they are rare.

Congenital rubella is the result of an infection in early pregnancy. The placenta and fetus become affected, resulting in serious abnormalities, the most common being defects of the heart and great vessels and deafness. Eye defects, such as cataract, glaucoma, and chorioretinitis, occur. Susceptibility to infection and abnormality of the immunoglobulins are typical.

Cultivation of the virus can be obtained in cell culture. Clinically, it propogates primarily in the cervical lymph nodes. After 7 days, viremia develops and lasts about 7 to 14 days. Symptomless viremia may be acquired during pregnancy and result in defects of the fetus. Lifelong immunity is acquired after one attack, and massive amounts of IgM antibodies are present.

There is no specific treatment. Because of the abnormalities occurring in the fetus, termination of pregnancy must be considered in the patient contracting rubella in early pregnancy.

NEWCASTLE DISEASE

This disease, discovered by Doyle in 1927 at Newcastle-upon-Tyne, is due to a virus of the paramyxovirus group and is a serious communicable disease of fowls causing economic disaster. The disease is found in poultry and in laboratory workers and veterinarians. Follicular conjunctivitis is the typical manifestation and is usually unilateral. The incubation period is 18 to 48 hours. The conjunctivitis is mild, with itching, and can be epidemic among poultry workers. The conjunctivitis often shows gelatinous swelling mainly on the lower lid, swelling of the preauricular glands, and mild systemic symptoms. This resolves rapidly in one or two days. Conjunctival hemorrhages can be present, but corneal complication is rare.

In laboratory study, cultivation is readily obtained in embryonated eggs and HeLa cell tissue culture. Basophilic cytoplasmic inclusion bodies can be demonstrated, and the specific antibodies determine the diagnosis.

Treatment is symptomatic.

MUMPS

Mumps (epidemic parotitis) is a contagious viral disease. Its viral origin was proven in 1934 by Johnson and Goodpasture. Epidemics of mumps are frequent, especially in military establishments. While the commonest manifestation is parotitis, other organs, such as the pancreas, ovaries, or testicles, may also be primarily affected. Hence, rather than "complications," the term "manifestations" is more accurate. Mumps is now regarded as a viremia rather than a localized infection of the salivary glands.

Many cases of ocular involvement have been reported.

Clinical Features. Diagnosis can be made upon the typical characteristics of clinical manifestations. The salivary gland's manifestations usually occur in children aged 5 to 13 years. The incubation period is 18 to 21 days, after which one or both parotids swell. There are accompanying fever and headache. Swelling of the submaxillary glands is often present. The portal of entry is usually the respiratory tract, but the conjunctival epithelium may be the primary site for multiplication of the virus. The virus may spread via the bloodstream, affecting certain parts of the body, including the eye, then symptoms appear. The disease may be complicated by generalized viremia and often by meningoencephalitis.

Mumps, while often symptomatic, may be symptomless.

Immunity is usually permanent after a single infection.

Findings in the Eye.   The complete review of ocular manifestations of the mumps virus is by Riffenburgh. Dacryoadenitis and optic neuritis most commonly occur. In epidemic mumps, dacryoadenitis may precede the parotitis (Galpine and Walkowski; Jones). The onset of dacryoadenitis is sudden, painful, and usually bilateral. Its duration is several weeks, and healing is without sequelae.

Optic neuritis or papillitis is usually benign, and only rarely does optic atrophy occur (Swab). Corneal infection is frequent, particularly during the febrile period (Danielson and Long). The most common corneal picture is an unusual unilateral interstitial keratitis (Nectoux). This keratitis is characterized by a dense opacity, which may rapidly progress to involve the entire cornea. Occasionally only one quadrant is affected. Numerous folds in Descemet's membrane are evident. The process disappears spontaneously, usually within two weeks, leaving no trace. This typical picture is regarded as pathognomonic for mumps. It may be associated with anterior uveitis. Occasionally a punctate ulcerative or nodular keratitis, resembling nummular keratitis, is seen. The other ocular manifestations, not infrequent, are conjunctivitis (usually without secretion), benign episcleritis, and scleritis (Kirber and Kirber).

Rare ocular manifestations are cortical blindness (Davis et al), central retinal vein occlusion and congenital abnormalities following mumps infection of the mother during the early months of pregnancy (Siegel and Greenberg).

Treatment.   The treatment is symptomatic. Concentrated normal gamma globulin has proved to be of no value, but the convalescent serum can be useful. Several steroid hormones have been used, but their value is not established.

MOLLUSCUM CONTAGIOSUM

Molluscum contagiosum was recognized as a clinical entity as early as 1817 (van Rooyen and Rhodes). It is common in Edinburgh, Scotland, but sporadic or epidemic occurrence is known in many parts of the world. The infection is spread by direct or indirect contact (eg, barbers, common towels, scratching). Swimming pools are one source of infection. Pigeons, dogs, and other domestic animals may develop molluscum and contaminate man.

Molluscum contagiosum is a local disease of mild infectivity. Its most interesting feature is the architecture of the molluscum body, once considered a protozoan parasite. These are now recognized as viral bodies, and study with the electron microscope has added knowledge of their detailed structure.

Clinical Features. Molluscum contagiosum is mainly a childhood disease, characterized by benign epithelial nodules on any part of the skin, especially the face. Mucous membranes of the genitalia are often involved. Lesions are uninflamed, round, waxy, and white. The summit is usually umbilicated, having a tiny black spot. Cheesy masses consisting of degenerated epithelial cells can readily be expressed. The typical lesions are easily diagnosed. However, sometimes they appear in atypical forms: sebaceous cyst, verruca, or milium (Curtin and Theodore).

Findings in the Eye. Ocular manifestation of molluscum contagiosum is primarily on the skin of the lid. The lesions vary in size from very small to giganteum (Meer Maastricht and Gomperts) and number from one to a dozen, sometimes grouped in semiconfluented masses. Suppuration due to secondary infection may occur. The lesions occasionally disappear spontaneously.

Various ocular manifestations due to extension of the skin molluscum have been described. Reviews of the literature are given by Duke-Elder, Lee, Magnus, Mather, and Rocha. If the lesion is situated at the lid margin (Plate 29, Fig. 1), conjunctivitis or keratitis or both may develop. Catarrhal conjunctivitis is usually a chronic, recurrent, or follicular type (Plate 29, Fig. 2) with considerable papillary hypertrophy and thickening of the conjunctiva, mainly on the upper lid. The picture resembles trachoma.

Several types of keratitis, independent or associated with the conjunctivitis, may develop: epithelial, punctate, marginal, or pannus. The pannus (Plate 29, Fig. 3) involves the upper part of the cornea and, together with follicular conjunctivitis, resembles the trachomatous process. The presence of molluscum contagiosum at the margin and the absence of trachomatous inclusion bodies are diagnostic aids. The complication disappears after removal of the lid lesion. Toxic or mechanical origin may therefore be considered. Nevertheless, direct viral invasion may occur as typical umbilicated nodules on the lower palpebral conjunctiva resembling chalazion or as conjunctival or corneal phlyctenulelike nodules.

Laboratory Studies. Numerous attempts to cultivate the virus have failed. Animal inoculation experiments have also been negative (Rake and Blank). Man is the only known host.

The virus is plentiful in individual skin lesions and can readily be demonstrated by the electron microscope (Banfield et al). This is one of the largest viruses, and its shape is ovoid.

The cytoplasmic, eosinophilic inclusion bodies, described by Henderson and by Paterson, were later shown to be composed of elementary bodies. Several stages of their development have been described. In the mature stage, the eosinophilic globular masses, separated by septa, represent aggregations of elementary bodies. The nucleus, pushed to the wall, becomes almost invisible (Plate 29, Fig. 4).

There is no evidence of immunity.

No specific treatment exists. Surgery is usually the best approach, although electrocoagulation may be preferred for lid margin lesions.

WARTS

Warts (verruca) are horny growths on the skin and, rarely, mucous membranes. They may occur as a primary invasion of the eye lids, particularly the lid margins. However, transmission from other body areas is a more common occurrence. Animals may be affected and can be a source of infection for man.

Thorough studies and references are given by Blank and Rake. Various clinical types, distinguished by structure, localization, age of patient, and other clinical features, are common warts (verruca vulgaris), flat warts (verruca plantaris), filiform warts (verruca filiformis), moist warts (venereal warts), and flat, greasy warts seen in the elderly (verruca senilis).

All warts are believed to be caused by a single virus, the human papovavirus. Verruca vulgaris, the most frequent type, is commonly seen in children. Girls are more subject to verruca plantaris than are boys or adults. Moist warts may be found on the conjunctiva, although they usually involve the genitalia. This type undergoes malignant changes more frequently than do the others. Filiform warts are the commonest warts of the lid skin and lid margins.

Like molluscum contagiosum, the wart virus is slow-growing and of mild infectivity. The incubation period is from 1 to 20 months. The infection is spread by direct or indirect contact (ie, barbers, common towels, shaking hands, communal washing facilities, bathing pools, or venereal contact). Warts are less common in the United States than in Europe. However, incidence is increasing in crowded military installations and in areas having poor hygiene.

Findings in the Eye. Filiform warts may involve the lid skin and are frequently associated with lesions of the bearded area, disseminated by shaving (Plate 29, Fig. 6). Rarely, cornu cutaneum (about 3 cm) at the inner lid canthus was observed by the author (Plate 29, Fig. 5).

Filiform and common warts, the most frequent lid margin warts, are slowly progressive. They may be single or coalescent and develop between the lashes, usually of the upper lids.

Conjunctivitis, keratitis, or even corneal ulceration may occasionally complicate lid margin warts. In contrast to molluscum contagiosum, the conjunctivitis is a subacute catarrhal type and is not follicular. Papillary hypertrophy of the conjunctiva is mostly at the inner angle and may be a manifestation of verruca. It sometimes has a raspberrylike appearance or appears as a soft peduncular growth with a tendency to recur. Duke-Elder has emphasized that the keratitis is strictly epithelial and often occurs without conjunctivitis. Considerable pain and photophobia are characteristic, and recurrence is frequent. A vascular type of keratitis somewhat like rosacea keratitis may occur. The exact mechanism of these complications is unknown. However, in analogy with molluscum contagiosum, a toxic, allergic, or mechanical origin may be assumed.

Additionally, it seems appropriate to mention the role of bacteria. The rough surface of the wart may become a locus for bacterial growth. Conjunctivitis or superficial keratitis can ensue from the infection itself or from bacterial sensitization.

Laboratory Studies.   Warts are infective, as proved in 1894 by inoculation of volunteers (Variot) and in 1907 by self-inoculation (Ciuffo). This was more fully confirmed and expanded by Wile and Kingery in 1919 and by Goodman and Greenwood in 1934. Practically all of the experimental work has been done with human volunteers. Numerous attempts to transmit warts to animals have failed or successful results have lacked confirmation. Growth has also failed in tissue culture.

Cytologic study in the past was confusing. The structures seen in the granular layer, such as keratohyaline granules, were once regarded as inclusion bodies. Later, the specific structures were recognized as the real inclusion bodies. Their positive Feulgen reaction confirms that they are newly formed DNA. The cells showing ballooning degeneration of the cytoplasm are called "bird's-eye cells." Studies with the electron microscope by Strauss et al and Melnick et al added significant knowledge concerning structure of the inclusion bodies, demonstrating a viral aggregation having the appearance of crystals.

An increased incidence of warts has been found in patients who have had kidney transplant and received immunosuppressive drugs.

Treatment.   There is no specific or uniform treatment. Every case must be individualized, although 0.7 percent solution of cantharon in equal parts of acetone and collodion often gives a good result (Book).

Surgical removal is often successful, although the lesion may recur on the scar. Chemical destruction is usually effective and simple. Trichloracetic acid, silver nitrate pencil, nitric acid, and salicylic acid have been successfully used.

Psychotherapy or suggestion therapy is widely accepted. Wart charmers use various mystical procedures (cited from Blank and Rake). An extensive review of psychotherapy was made by Allington in 1952. Many agree that none of the chemical and physical methods are better than suggestion.

Spontaneous disappearance of warts has been observed.

REFERENCES

General, Variola and Vaccinia

Buddingh GJ: Infection of the chorio-allantois of the chick embryo as a diagnostic test for variola. Am J Hyg 28:130, 1938

Chapin CV, Smith JJ: Permanency of mild type of smallpox. Prev Med 6:273, 1932

Duke-Elder WS: Text-book of Ophthalmology. St. Louis, Mosby, 1965, vol 8

Groffead GW, Harrison SW: Vaccinia conjunctivitis. Am J Ophthalmol 53:531, 1962

Isaacs A: Interferon. Sci Am 240:51, 1961

Laurance B, Cunliffe AC, Dudgeon JA: Vaccinia gangrenosa. The report of a case of prolonged generalized vaccinia. Arch Dis Child 27:482, 1952

Lazarus AS, Eddie B, Meyer KF: Propagation of variola virus in the developing egg. Proc Soc Exp Biol Med 36:7, 1937

Perera CA: Vaccinal disciform keratitis following accidental inoculation of the eyelid. Arch Ophthalmol 24:352, 1940

Rosen E: The significance of ocular complications following vaccination. Br J Ophthalmol 33:358, 1949

Saxena RC, Gang KC, Ramchand S: Ankyloblepharom following smallpox. Am J Ophthalmol 61:169, 1966

Sommerville J, Napier W, Dick A: Kaposi's varicelliform eruption: record of an outbreak. Br J Dermatol 63:203, 1951

Stanley WM, Valens EG: Viruses and the Nature of Life. New York, Dutton, 1961

van Rooyen CE, Rhodes AJ: Virus Diseases of Man. New York, Nelson, 1948, chap 26–35

Herpesvirus simplex

Andrews CH, Carmichael EA: A note on the presence of antibodies to herpes virus in post-encephalitic and other human sera. Lancet 1:857, 1930

Braley AE: Acute herpetic keratoconjunctivitis. Am J Ophthalmol 43 (Part 2): 105, 1957

Buddingh GJ, Schrum DI, Lanier JC, Guidry DJ: Studies of the natural history of herpes simplex infections. Pediatrics 11:595, 1953

Carroll JM, Matrda J, Laibson P et al: Recurrence of herpetic keratitis following iodoxuridine therapy. Am J Ophthalmol 63:103, 1967

Cavara V, Di Ferdinando R: Sympathetic ophthalmia and herpetic infection (abstract). Am J Ophthalmol 32:1313, 1949

Cibis A, Burde RM: Herpes simplex virus-induced congenital cataracts. Arch Ophthalmol 85:220, 1971

Cogan DG, Kuwabara T, Young F et al: Herpes simplex retinopathy in an infant. Arch Ophthalmol 72:641, 1964

Coons AH, Creech HJ, Jones RN: Immunological properties of antibody containing a fluorescent group. Proc Soc Exp Biol Med 47:200, 1941

Deutsch FH: Recurrent herpes simplex keratitis treated with hormone-induced amenorrhea. Am J Ophthalmol 61:1527, 1966

Doane F, Rhodes AY, Ormsby HL: Tissue culture techniques in the study of herpetic infections of the eye. Am J Ophthalmol 40 (Part 2):189, 1957

Font RL: Chronic ulcerative keratitis caused by herpes simplex virus. Arch Ophthalmol 90:382, 1973

Gallardo E: Primary herpes simplex keratitis; clinical and experimental study. Arch Ophthalmol 30:217, 1943

Hagler WS, Walters P, Nahmias A et al: Ocular involvement in neonatal herpes simplex virus infection. Arch Ophthalmol 82:169, 1969

Hanna L, Jawetz E, Coleman VR: The significance of isolating herpes simplex virus from the eye. Am J Ophthalmol 43 (Part 2):126, 1957

Hogan MJ: Corneal transplantation in the treatment of herpetic disease of the cornea. Am J Ophthalmol 43 (Part 2):147, 1957

Hogan MJ, Kimura SJ, Thygeson P: Pathology of herpes simplex keratitis. Am J Ophthalmol 57:551, 1964

Howard GM, Kaufman HE: Herpes simplex keratitis. Special reviews. Arch Ophthalmol 67:373, 1962

Howard RO: Herpes simplex keratoconjunctivitis. Am J Ophthalmol 62:907, 1966

Hughes WF: Treatment of herpes simplex keratitis. Am J Ophthalmol 67:313, 1969

Hutchison DS, Smith R, Haughton P et al: Congenital herpetic keratitis. Arch Ophthalmol 93:70, 1975

Kaufman HE, Brown D, Ellison E et al: Herpes virus in the lacrimal gland, conjunctiva and cornea of man: a chronic infection. Am J Ophthalmol 65:32, 1968

Kaufman HE, Ellison E, Waltman S et al: Double-stranded RNA and interferon-induced in herpes simplex keratitis. Am J Ophthalmol 68:486, 1969

Kaufman HE, Nesburn AB, Maloney ED: IDU therapy of herpes simplex. Arch Ophthalmol 67:583, 1962

Kiffney GT Jr: Linear endothelial vesicles or herpes corneae posterior. Am J Ophthalmol 59:466, 1965

Kimura SJ, Okumoto MA: The effect of corticosteroids on experimental herpes simplex keratoconjunctivitis in the rabbit. Am J Ophthalmol 43 (Part 2):107, 1957

Langston RHS, Pavan-Langston D, Dohlman CH: Antiviral medication and corneal wound healing. Arch Ophthalmol 92:509, 1974

Lennette EH, van Allen A: Laboratory diagnosis of herpetic infections of the eye. Am J Ophthalmol 43 (Part 2):118, 1957

Metcalf J, Kaufman H: Herpetic stromal keratitis. Am J Ophthalmol 82:827, 1976

Oh JO, Kimura S, Ostler H et al: Acute ocular infection by Type 2 herpes simplex virus in adults. Arch Ophthalmol 93:1127, 1975

Oh JO, Stevens TR: I. Comparison of Types 1 and 2 herpes virus hominis infection of rabbit eyes. Arch Ophthalmol 90:473, 1973

Ormsby HL: Superficial forms of herpetic keratitis. Am J Ophthalmol 43 (Part 2):107, 1957

Pavan-Langston D, Langston R, Geary P: Prophylaxis and therapy of experimental ocular herpes simplex. Arch Ophthalmol 92:417, 1974

Peister R, Richards J, Dohlman C: Recurrence of herpetic keratitis in corneal grafts. Am J Ophthalmol 73:192, 1972

Rake GW: The etiologic role of the virus of herpes simplex in ophthalmic disease. Am J Ophthalmol 43 (Part 2):113, 1957

Scott TFM, Coriell LL, Blank H, Gray A: The growth curve of the virus of herpes simplex on the chorioallantoic membrane of the embryonated hen's egg. J Immunol 71:134, 1953

Stevens TR, Oh JO: II. Histopathologic and virologic studies. Arch Ophthalmol 90:477, 1973

Tanaka N, Kimura SJ: Localization of herpes simplex antigen and virus. Arch Ophthalmol 78:68, 1967

Thomas CI: The Cornea. Springfield, Ill, Thomas, 1955

Thygeson P, Hogan MJ, Kimura SJ: Cortisone and hydrocortisone in ocular infections. Trans Am Acad Ophthalmol 57:64, 1953

Thygeson P, Kimura SJ: Deep forms of herpetic keratitis. Am J Ophthalmol 43 (Part 2):109, 1957

Thygeson P, Kimura SJ, Hogan MJ: Observations on herpetic keratitis and keratoconjunctivitis. Arch Ophthalmol 56:375, 1956

Wilkie JS, et al: Credé prophylaxis and neonatal corneal infection with herpes virus. Arch Ophthalmol 91:386, 1974

Varicella-Zoster Group

Blodi FC: Ophthalmic zoster in malignant disease. Am J Ophthalmol 65:686, 1968

Bonzas A: Canalicular inflammation in ophthalmic cases of H. zoster and simplex. Am J Ophthalmol 60:713, 1965

Goodpasture EW, Anderson K: Infection of human skin, grafted on the chorioallantois of chick embryos, with the virus of herpes zoster. Am J Pathol 20:447, 1944

Haggerty RJ, Eley RC: Varicella and cortisone (Letter to Editor). Pediatrics 18:160, 1956

Hayashi K, Uchida Y, Ohshima M et al: Fluorescent antibody study of Herpes zoster keratitis. Am J Ophthalmol 75:795, 1973

Kielar R, Cunningham G, Gerson K: Occurrence of herpes zoster in child with absent immunoglobulin "G" and deficiency of delayed hypersensitivity. Am J Ophthalmol 27:555, 1971

Klein BA, Farkas TG: Pseudomelanoma of the iris after H. zoster ophthalmicus. Am J Ophthalmol 57:392, 1964

Marsh RJ: Herpes zoster keratitis. Trans Ophthalmol Soc UK 93:181, 1973

Pavan-Langston D, McCulley JP: Herpes zoster dendritic keratitis. Arch Ophthalmol 89:25, 1973

Pemberton JW: Optic atrophy in herpes zoster ophthalmicus. Am J Ophthalmol 58:852, 1964

Piebenga LW, Laibson PR: Dendritic lesions in herpes zoster ophthalmicus. Arch Ophthalmol 90:268, 1973

Rogers JW: Internal ophthalmoplegia following chickenpox. Arch Ophthalmol 71:617, 1964

Scheie HG: Herpes zoster ophthalmicus. Trans Ophthalmol Soc UK 90:899, 1970

Steiner G: Zur Inokulation vericellen. Wien Med Wochnschr 25:306, 1875

Weller TH: Serial propagation in vitro of agents producing inclusion bodies derived from varicella and herpes zoster. Proc Soc Exp Biol Med 83:340, 1953

Weller TH, Coons AH: Fluorescent antibody studies with agents of varicella and herpes zoster propagated in vitro. Proc Soc Exp Biol Med 86:789, 1954

Adenovirus Group

Burn R, Potter M: Epidemic keratoconjunctivitis due to adenovirus 19. Am J Ophthalmol 81:27, 1976

Dawson CR, Hanna L, Togni B: Adenovirus type 8 infection in the United States. Arch Ophthalmol 87:258, 1972

Enders JF, Bell JA, Dingle JH, et al: "Adenoviruses": Group name proposed for new respiratory-tract viruses. Science 124:119, 1956

Golden B, et al: Epidemic keratoconjunctivitis: a new approach. Trans Am Acad Ophthalmol Otolaryngol 75:1216, 1971

Green J, Hung T, Sung S: Neurologic complication with elevated antibody titre after acute hemorrhagic conjunctivitis. Am J Ophthalmol 80:832, 1975

Hilleman MR, Werner JH: Recovery of new agent from patients with acute respiratory illness. Proc Soc Exp Biol Med 85:183, 1954

Huebner RJ, Rowe WP, Ward TG, Parrott RH, Bell JA: Adenoidal-pharyngeal-conjunctival agents. A newly recognized group of common viruses of the respiratory system. N Engl J Med 251:1077, 1954

Jawetz E, Hanna L, Kimura SJ, Thygeson P: A new type of APC virus from follicular conjunctivitis. Am J Ophthalmol 41:231, 1956

Jawetz E, Kimura S, Nicholas AN, Thygeson P, Hanna L: New type of APC virus from epidemic keratoconjunctivitis. Science 122:1190, 1955

Jones BR: Epidemic haemorrhagic conjunctivitis in London, 1971. A conjunctiva picornavirus infection. Trans Ophthalmol Soc UK 92:625, 1972

Kimura SJ, Hanna MA, Nicholas BA, Thygeson P, Jawetz E: Sporadic cases of pharyngoconjunctival fever in northern California, 1955–1956. Am J Ophthalmol 43 (Part 2):14, 1957

Laibson PR, Green WR: Conjunctival membranes in epidemic keratoconjunctivitis. Arch Ophthalmol 83:100, 1970

Laibson PR, Ortolam G, Dupre S: Community and hospital outbreak of epidemic keratoconjunctivitis. Arch Ophthalmol 80:467, 1968

Laibson PR, et al: Corneal infiltrates in epidemic keratoconjunctivitis. Arch Ophthalmol 84:36, 1970

Mitsui Y, Hanabusa J, Minoda R, Ogata S: Effect of inoculating adenovirus (APC virus) type 8 into human volunteers. Am J Ophthalmol 43 (Part 2):84, 1957

Mitsui Y, Jawetz E: Isolation of adenovirus type 8 (APC type 8) from a case of epidemic keratoconjunctivitis in Japan. Am J Ophthalmol 43 (Part 2):91, 1957

O'Day D, Guyer B, Hierholzer J et al: Clinical and laboratory evaluation of EKC due to adenovirus type 8 and 19. Am J Ophthalmol 81:207, 1976

Rivers TM, Horsfall FL: Viral and Rickettsial Infections of Man, 3rd ed. Philadelphia, Lippincott, 1959

Rose HM (ed): Viral Infections of Infancy and Childhood. New York, Hoeber, 1960

Rowe WP, Huebner RJ, Gilmore LK, Parrott RH, Ward TG: Isolation of a cytopathic agent from human adenoids undergoing spontaneous degenerations in tissue culture. Proc Soc Exp Biol Med 84:570, 1953

Tanaka C: Epidemic keratoconjunctivitis in Japan and the Orient. Paper given at Keratoconjunctivitis Symposium, San Francisco, Sept 7–8, 1956

Thygeson P: Office and dispensary transmissions of epidemic keratoconjunctivitis. Am J Ophthalmol 43 (Part 2):98, 1957

Ward TG, Huebner RJ, Rowe WP, Ryan RW, Bell JA: Production of pharyngoconjunctival fever in human volunteers inoculated with APC viruses. Science 122:1086, 1955

Measles, Rubella, Newcastle Disease

Anderson JF, Goldberger J: Experimental measles in the monkey: a supplemental note. Public Health Rep 26:887, 1911

Blank H, Rake G: Viral and Rickettsial Diseases of the Skin, Eye and Mucous Membranes of Man. Boston, Little, Brown, 1955.

Duke-Elder WS: Text-book of Ophthalmology. St. Louis, Mosby, 1965, vol 8; p 334

Rake G, Shaffer MF: Propagation of the agent of measles in the fertile hen's egg. Nature 144:672, 1939

Mumps

Danielson RW, Long JC: Keratitis due to mumps. Am J Ophthalmol 24:655, 1942

Davis LE, Harris A, Chin T et al: Transient cortical blindness and ataxia associated with mumps. Arch Ophthalmol 85:366, 1971

Galpine JF, Walkowski J: A case of mumps with involvement of the lacrimal glands. Br Med J 1:1069, 1952

Jones BR: Clinical features and aetiology of dacryoadenitis. Trans Ophthalmol Soc UK 75:435, 1955

Kirber MW, Kirber HP: Factors influencing the course of experimental eye infection with mumps. Am J Ophthalmol 57:600, 1964

Nectoux R: Keratite ourlienne. Ann Ocul 179:597, 1946

Riffenburgh RD: Ocular manifestations of mumps. Special reviews. Arch Ophthalmol 66:739, 1961

Siegel M, Greenberg M: Virus diseases in pregnancy and their effects on the fetus. Am J Ophthalmol 66:739, 1961

Swab CM: Encephalitic optic neuritis and atrophy due to mumps. Arch Ophthalmol 19:926, 1938

Molluscum Contagiosum, Warts

Allington HV: Review of the psychotherapy of warts. Arch Dermatol 66:316, 1952

Banfield WG, Bunting H, Strauss MJ, Melnick JL: Electronmicrographs of thin sections of molluscum contagiosum. Proc Soc Exp Biol Med 77:843, 1951

Blank H, Rake G: Viral and Rickettsial Diseases of the Skin, Eye and Mucous Membranes of Man. Boston, Little, Brown, 1955

Book RH: Treatment of palpebral warts with cantharon. Am J Ophthalmol 60:259, 1965

Ciuffo G: Innesto positivo con filtrato di verruca volgare. G Ital Mal Ven 48:12, 1907

Curtin BJ, Theodore FH: Ocular molluscum contagiosum. Am J Ophthalmol 39:302, 1955

Duke-Elder WS: Text-book of Ophthalmology. St. Louis, Mosby, 1965, vol 8, p 376

Goodman J Jr, Greenwood AM: Verrucae, a review. Arch Dermatol 30:659, 1934

Henderson W: Edinburgh Med Surg J 56:213, 1841

Lee OS Jr: Keratitis occurring with molluscum contagiosum. Arch Ophthalmol 31:64, 1944

Magnus JA: Unilateral follicular conjunctivitis due to molluscum contagiosum. Br J Ophthalmol 28:245, 1944

Mathur SP: Ocular complications in molluscum contagiosum. Br J Ophthalmol 44:572, 1960

Meer Maastricht BCJvd, Gomperts CE: Molluscum contagiosum giganteum. Am J Ophtalmol 33:965, 1950

Melnick JL, Bunting H, Banfield WG, Strauss MJ, Gaylord WH: Electron microscopy of viruses of human papilloma molluscum contagiosum and vaccinia, including observations on the formation of virus within the cells. Ann NY Acad Sci 54:1214, 1952

Paterson R: Edinburgh Med Surg J 56:279, 1841

Rake G, Blank H: The relationship of host and virus in molluscum contagiosum. J Invest Dermatol 15:81, 1950

Rocha H: Molluscum contagiosum (abstract). Am J Ophthalmol 27:929, 1944

Strauss MJ, Bunting H, Melnick JL: Viruslike particles and inclusion bodies in skin papillomas. J Invest Dermatol 15:433, 1950

van Rooyen CE, Rhodes AJ: Virus Diseases of Man, 2nd ed. New York, Nelson, 1948

Variot G: Un cas d'inoculation experimentale des verrues de l'enfant a l'homme. J Clin Ther Inf (Paris) 2:529, 1894

Wile UJ, Kingery LB: The etiology of common warts. JAMA 73:970, 1919

4

Fungi

The incidence of fungal infections has a geographic distribution. They are most common in tropical countries. In India mycotic infections are a big problem. They are also frequently found in Florida largely among the agricultural population. Fungal infection has increased sharply in the west, probably due to two main factors: the disturbance in the balance of the normal flora by antibiotic usage and the alteration in the resistance of host tissue, a result of the topical use of corticosteroids.

Fungi are important both as vectors of disease and as agents for industrial fermentation. They are vegetable organisms of low order and are structurally more complicated than bacteria, being larger, vacuolized, and usually having a sexual mechanism. Lacking chlorophyll, they are not photosynthetic. The soil is their most common environment, and they are a leading cause of plant disease.

Many of the fungi which act as laboratory contaminants were once considered nonpathogenic. Recent studies reveal that some of these so-called nonpathogenic fungi may cause severe, even fatal, diseases in man (Francois, Birge). They are mostly imperfect fungi because of their asexual spores. The type of mycosis and its distribution vary geographically.

Mycotic diseases, including those of the eye, appear to be on the rise since the advent of antibiotics and steroids (Mitsui et al; Thygeson) and the increased therapeutic use of antimetabolic drugs.

As descriptions of fungi are complex and specialized, the ophthalmologist need not be acquainted with a detailed study. Only the practical general aspects will be discussed herein.

Morphology. Fungi are usually multicellular, filamentous structures, although yeasts and some branched fungi are unicellular. A hypha is an individual filament, which may divide by the septum (sep-

228

tate hyphae). A mass of hyphae constitute the mycelium, which is better demonstrated in culture. Mycelia can also be shown in superficial mycoses of the skin or mucous membranes.

Fungi are gram-positive. Some are acid-fast and can be mistaken for tubercle bacilli. Staining is usually uneven, creating a granular appearance. Most fungi possess cell walls and vacuoles, and special staining demonstrates these. The filaments of some fungi fragment easily into bacillary and coccoid elements.

Microscopic examination of original clinical material is important and may lead to diagnosis of mycosis more readily than the culturing.

Culture. Fungi grow readily on most routine laboratory media aerobically and at room temperature. Corneal and conjunctival scrapings and swab specimens can be used for culture on blood agar, thyloglycollate broth, Sabouraud's medium, and liquid shake-culture, the latter being preferable to solid media, particularly in a small inoculum, eg, from a corneal ulcer. After primary isolation identification is necessary. On media, fungal growth is slow, usually taking more than one week. The culture must be prevented from drying. Sabouraud's medium is the most satisfactory for fungi. However, special media and methods are needed to identify certain species. The cultures show a great variation of appearance, even on the same medium, and identification is not easy. The filamentous colonies are usually powdery, cottony, prickly, or with a leathery consistency. The growth has a marked tendency to spread over the surface of the medium.

Yeast colonies are soft and bacterialike, consisting only of budding cells (eg, *Cryptococcus*). Yeastlike colonies are also soft, but besides the budding cells on the surface of the medium, there are hyphae which penetrate it (eg, in *Candida* species).

Examination of the Fungi. Fungi are identified on the basis of the type of spores and their arrangement. Several special methods are used to prepare specimens for spore examination. For some species, the tube or plate is placed on the stage and examined, using the low-power objective (Smolin and Okumoto). This must be done carefully without disturbing the growth, and the hyphae and spores can be seen. There are two types of hyphae: vegetative, to secure food, and fertile, to produce spores.

Skin, hair, and nails should be examined on a slide with a drop of 10 percent potassium hydroxide. It is best to heat the slide before examination in order to clarify the specimen. Exudates or other direct specimens are usually examined as fresh preparations or may be stained by various methods.

Laboratory diagnosis in fungal keratitis has been studied comprehensively by Wilson and Sexton. Corneal scraping is most important for initial diagnosis and must be done correctly. The necrotic mass must first be removed, then the scrapings are taken from the center of the cornea as deeply as possible. The specimen must be used for at least three slides: (1) for wet preparation, (2) for gram-stain, and (3) for Giemsa stain. Gram stain may well demonstrate yeast cells. Giemsa stain and PAS technique can be of considerable value in identifying both yeast and hyphae.

The wet preparation is examined classically by adding a small drop of 10 or 20 percent aqueous solution of potassium hydroxide to the slide, covering with a coverglass, and studying it microscopically. The hyphae (septate or nonseptate) can be demonstrated. In cases of endophthalmitis the specimen must be taken by the aspiration method. The same procedure as that for examination of a specimen from the cornea is followed. Fluorescent microscopy has been studied as a promising new technique.

Extreme caution should be taken in working with cultures, as several fatal infections by spores or mycelia have been reported in laboratory workers. Cultures, being puffy or powdery, contaminate the air, and workers can be invaded by inhaling the powder. Therefore, the plate containing the fungus should be placed on a dampened cloth during examination and must be opened carefully. From the culture some filamentous fungi are examined in a drop of mounting medium on the slide. The filaments must be carefully teased with needles, then covered with a coverglass. Lactophenol cotton blue, glycerin, or eosin can be used as a mounting medium. The yeastlike colonies are best examined by emulsifying a bit of the colony in a drop of water and preparing the usual wet slide.

Reproduction. Fungi reproduce by the formation of spores (blastospore, chlamydospore, arthrospore, and conidia), usually by a sexual mechanism (the reproduction of yeasts is asexual only—they multiply by budding). Multiplication of mycelial fungi is mainly apical on the aerial mycelium.

There are two main types of spores: ascospores (sexual spores), which develop from special cells in the mycelium by nuclear fusion, and thallospores (asexual spores), formed by segmentation of the hypha. Thallospores may develop a thick protective wall and are then called "chlamydospores." Many other types of spores are designated.

Serologic Characteristics. Some fungi show agglutination or complement-fixation reactions and various phenomena of immunity and hypersensitivity. Recently, serologic typing according to capsular material (carbohydrates, polysaccharides, and proteins) has been used for diagnosis of some mycoses. A delayed tuberculinlike skin test is diagnostically important in many mycoses.

Pathogenesis and Pathology.   Three important factors must be considered in the pathogenesis and pathology of mycoses: endotoxin, multiplication of the fungi (usually very slow), and the phenomenon of hypersensitivity. The mycotic infections are chiefly chronic and vary in severity. They may be extremely mild; in mycosis of the skin, hair, and nails the fungi are almost saprophytic and behave as foreign bodies. In some other cases, mycotic diseases are generalized and even fatal (deep mycosis). Fungi do not usually produce epidemics. Mycoses are said to be found more frequently in males than in females (Nema et al; Olson).

It has been reported that normal flora from the conjunctiva and lid margins was positive for fungi in a high percentage of those tested (Tomar et al; Fazakas; Olson; Wilson et al), the most common fungus present being *Aspergillus. Penicillium, Aspergillus, Alternaria, Cephalosporium,* and particularly *Fusarium* are most common in southern countries.

In mycoses, any pathologic process may occur, such as suppuration (resembling staphylococcal infection) or caseous necrosis with resultant fibrosis. These may be mistaken for tuberculosis. Some mycoses resemble cancer. Tuberclelike giant cell granuloma is the most typical finding in mycosis. In this, the phagocytosis of fungi by reticuloendothelial cells may remind one of storage.

Hypersensitivity reactions occur frequently in mycoses, giving a valuable diagnostic indication (Henly et al; Simon).

Intravenous inoculation of rabbits or intraperitoneal injection of guinea pigs with fungal culture is often used to determine the pathogenicity of fungi.

In almost all mycoses, there is a history of injury to the host preceding invasion by the fungus. The predisposing factors are previous trauma particularly people like farmers who work with vegetables, diseases such as *Herpesvirus simplex* infection, keratoconjunctivitis sicca, exposure keratitis, and previous treatment with cortisone and antibiotics.

Polymorphism is a typical feature of fungi. Their morphologic and biologic characteristics are not constant. Hence, the classification is complex and confusing. In medical practice, the most convenient division of fungi is based on the anatomic location of the mycotic lesions. Two groups are distinguished: deep mycoses, chiefly with systemic involvement, and superficial mycoses, extremely rarely affecting the general health. The eye can be involved secondarily to systemic mycosis, by continuation from surrounding areas, or by metastasis from distant organs.

Postoperative fungal endophthalmitis has increased. Endophthalmitis was reported in a patient having a filtering bleb while wearing contact lenses (Ashine and Ellis). There has also been an increase in keratitis. Diagnosis of fungal keratitis is frequently unsatisfactory. Kaufman and Wood summarized its typical clinical features as follows: (1) the presence of Descemet's folds in superficial keratitis, (2) hyphate ulcer (branching lines in the corneal stroma), (3) satellite lesions, and (4) hypopyon in small central ulcers. Histopathologic findings by Naumann et al showed that in 73 cases, fungus was found typically in the deep parenchyma and was conspicuously absent on the surface. Hyphae are distributed parallel to the corneal lamella and found beyond the area of clinical signs. Therefore, negative smear and culture do not rule out the presence of fungi, which are often found only in section.

There have been findings of fungal contaminants associated with the wearing of soft contact lenses (Brown). Most unusual was the invasion of such lenses by fungi, diagnosed in section (Palmer et al). Boiling the lenses is the most effective method of asepsis, although high temperatures may lead to deterioration of the lenses.

Treatment.   Antifungal drugs, such as nystatin, amphoteracin B, pimaricine, and many others named by Jones, may be effective but only in certain infections, and they are not always successful. The best results are obtained from combined treatment with antifungal drugs and surgery (Polack et al). Penetrating keratoplasty gives a good result, as does conjunctival flap.

In any treatment of keratomycosis, previous debridement is necessary. Experimental antilymphatic serum (ALS) has been used effectively (Joklik) alone and in combination with steroids in order to suppress delayed hypersensitivity.

In the opinion of the majority, steroids are contraindicated in fungal infection. Thygeson was the first to report in his experimental work that corticosteroids greatly facilitated the development of mycotic keratitis.

ACTINOMYCES AND LEPTOTHRIX

Actinomyces were once regarded as true fungi. Now, many consider them filamentous bacteria, while others regard them as midway between fungi and bacteria. The genera *Actinomyces* and *Nocardia* are important in human pathology. Both these genera are in the order Actinomycetales. In the 8th edition of *Bergey's Manual*, *Actinomyces* is classified as a species in the family Actinomycetaceae, and *Nocardia* is in the family Nocardiaceae. The genus *Actinomyces* is mainly composed of facultative anaerobes, and *Nocardia* of obligate aerobes.

Actinomyces

Actinomyces species cause actinomycosis. The species *Actinomyces bovis* infects cattle, and the species *Actinomyces israelii* affects man. However, saprophytic species of *Actinomyces* predominate, being found on grain, grass, or water. Many varieties, including pathogenic ones, are present in the human teeth, tonsils, or pharynx.

Morphology.   These organisms are long filaments or rods with clubbed ends. They stain gram-positive (non-acid-fast), resembling corynebacteria in their irregular staining, arrangement, and club shape. Some filaments have false branching, and true branching is uncommon. Later, the filaments undergo segmentation into rods, which are often clubbed, or into coccoid bodies, which are regarded as spores.

Culture.   Species of *Actinomyces* grow anaerobically and slowly, taking two weeks or more. Thioglycollate is a satisfactory liquid medium, showing a growth of fluffy balls. Blood dextrose agar in shake culture may be used (Sabouraud's agar will not support these organisms). The colonies are small, irregular, grayish or white, and their rough surface appears nodular. Most strains are nonhemolytic and nonproteolytic. In smears from a colony, long, branching filaments are seen.

Staphylococci are usually present in the culture as secondary invaders.

Pathology.   Actinomycosis may be localized or generalized, and it tends toward chronicity. The process, often preceded by trauma, involves mainly the face or neck, less often the lungs or abdomen. Nodules, with central caseation surrounded by granulomatous tissue, are typical. They frequently become abscessed. Tissue sections under the microscope show small, round, yellow granules called "Drusen," each of which consists of a mass of branching filaments. They are the best material for laboratory diagnosis. Because of their color, Drusen are sometimes rather confusingly designated "sulfur granules." The periphery of a Drusen is surrounded by radiating clubs, whence originated the now seldom-used term "ray fungus" for *Actinomyces*.

Hypersensitivity to *Actinomyces* is a frequent phenomenon.

Findings in the Eye.   Involvement of the eyelids, though infrequent, usually occurs by contiguous spread from adjacent parts of the face or sinuses. The infection is occasionally primary. Indolent subcutaneous nodules develop. Usually multiple, they become interconnected, causing a honeycomb appearance. Spreading to the surface of the skin, the nodules break down, and a purulent discharge follows, which contains yellowish or greenish Drusen.

Actinomycosis may also involve the lid margins, causing many small, indolent abscesses with a tendency to ulcerate.

An exudative, purulent conjunctivitis may occur, particularly in children. In adults, it is mostly secondary to canaliculitis, although it can be primary and is associated with swelling of the preauricular glands. The painless and freely movable nodules sometimes occur on the bulbar conjunctiva, near the limbus. Their association with blepharoconjunctivitis has been observed.

Intraocular infection, metastatic (Verhoeff) or following cataract extraction, and infection of the orbit from surrounding infected sinuses have been reported. A corneal ulcer of considerable severity was observed. It was torpid, gray or yellowish in color, surrounded by a yellow gutter of demarcation, and associated with iritis and hypopyon.

In severe ring abscess the entire cornea can be involved within 24 hours. Superficial punctate keratitis with tiny, yellowish lesions and pannus may occur.

Painless nodules or abscesses in deep tissue often result in fistulas, and the presence of Drusen is characteristic. The clinical picture is not always pathognomonic, and microscopic diagnosis, particularly of the granules, is most important.

Streptothrix. The historic background of *Streptothrix* has been given by Pine et al. More than 100 years have passed since von Graefe established the fungal etiology of the concretions in the lacrimal canal. At that time, the species of fungus was not identified. In 1875, the name *Streptothrix* was given to it by Cohn. Since the condition is rare and cultivation of the organism is difficult, its identification is not yet established. The name *Streptothrix* has usually been used on the basis of clinical features, being almost pathognomonic for concretions in the canaliculus (Bruce; Elliot; Ellis; Nagel; Theodore). Recently, various other genera *(Candida, Nocardia, Actinomyces)* have been identified as causes of lacrimal concretions. Therefore the question persists concerning the identification of *Streptothrix.*

Several investigators established *Streptothrix* as anaerobic *Actinomyces,* and, even recently, the term was used as a synonym for both aerobic and anaerobic *Actinomyces.* The classification remains to be fully clarified. Some general bacteriologists propose that the name *Streptothrix* be abandoned, but in ophthalmology this name is widely accepted.

It seems advisable for clinicians to use the term "concretions of the canaliculi" or "canaliculitis" instead of streptothricosis. Identification of the organism is important for further clarification of nomenclature.

MORPHOLOGY. *Streptothrix* (actinomyces) is studied in material obtained from the concretions of canaliculitis. The concretion must be squeezed and crushed on a slide. Saline solution is added to this very dry material, then the preparation is gram-stained. In our laboratory we have found that Giemsa staining reveals the structure more distinctly. The organisms are branched filaments which readily segment into rods and coccoid forms (Plate 30, Fig. 4). Staining by the gram stain varies. Some bacillary forms are gram-negative. According to Ellis et al, the gram-positive coccoid forms, which they call "streptococci," are actually arthrospores or oidiospores. Because of the polymorphic appearance in smears, *Streptothrix* can easily be confused with bacteria, and bacterial secondary invaders are always present in the concretions. All this must be thoroughly considered, since diagnosis is usually determined by microscopic examination of original smears.

CULTIVATION. The cultivation of *Streptothrix* (actinomyces) is difficult because the organism is anaerobic, and the concretions usually contain numerous secondary bacterial invaders. However, the organisms are successfully cultivated in Brewer's medium in an anaerobic zone of the tube. Growth requires about nine days and consists mainly of a mass of hyphae, chains of cocci, and bacilli.

FINDINGS IN THE EYE. *Streptothrix* is the almost exclusive etiologic agent of mycotic canaliculitis. Other ocular manifestations of *Streptothrix* mycosis are rare. Mycotic canaliculitis is practically restricted to women. It is usually unilateral, the lower canaliculus being chiefly involved (Plate 30, Fig. 1). Initially, lacrimation is the only symptom, and the process can be easily overlooked. Later, a characteristic localized swelling develops in the area of the canaliculus. An accumulation of concretions causes the swelling, but local inflammation is mild. The related punctum lacrimalis becomes dilated, and later a chronic, stubborn unilateral conjunctivitis, sometimes with copious yellowish or greenish discharge, occurs.

The concretions needed for diagnostic examination should be expressed by careful squeezing. Put any suitable hard support behind the canaliculus and press. Sometimes the canaliculus has to be split to obtain the concretions. According to their age, the color varies from gray to yellow to brown. Microscopically, a concretion consists of a mass of branching filaments, spores, and varying bacteria (Plate 30, Fig. 4).

Treatment. This requires complete removal of the concretions. Curettage, the simplest method, is usually preceded by splitting the canaliculus through the punctum. The procedure must be done thoroughly, but gently, to prevent recurrence and spreading of the infection. The treatment is completed by instillation of a 1 percent solution of tincture of iodine or a solution of penicillin. Sulfonamide or penicillin and other antibiotics can be effective, but treatment must be prolonged.

Nocardia

The genus *Nocardia* includes many species living free in nature. *Nocardia asteroides* has been found to be a human pathogen.

Morphology. *Nocardia* shows branching filaments, some of which have a tendency to fragment into rods and cocci. All of the species stain gram-positive. Some are also acid-fast and may be mistaken for the tubercle bacillus.

Yellowish, red, or brown mycelial granules, consisting of the organisms, may be seen in the pus. This is the best specimen for laboratory examination.

Culture. *Nocardia* grows readily on a variety of simple media, at room temperature. Sabouraud's medium is usually used; on this, growth takes three to four weeks. On simple media the growth is even slower. The colonies are wrinkled and crumbling, resembling those of mycobacteria (Plate 30, Fig. 3). However, a great variation in the appearance of the cultures, even on the same medium, is typical. Some colonies produce aerial mycelia, which have a chalky and powdery appearance. The color of the colonies may differ, being creamy, yellow, pink, or red.

Pathology. Nocardiosis is a chronic, suppurative process associated with granuloma (mycetoma) and draining sinuses. The pus usually contains granules consisting of *Nocardia* organisms. The process is found chiefly in bones and is characterized by multiple lesions, followed by drainage. After months or even years, deformities, particularly of the foot (madura foot), ensue. *Nocardia* contaminates wounds, causing localized mycetoma. When inhaled, the organism may cause pulmonary disease, usually manifested as tuberculosislike infection. A similar process may occur in the brain.

Nocardiosis may remain localized or become generalized by metastasis.

Findings in the Eye. Little has been published about ocular nocardiosis. Chronic keratoconjunctivitis may occur secondarily to nocardiosis of adjacent areas. *N. asteroides* infection of the lacrimal duct has been reported by Penikett and Rees.

Schardt et al have described a case of a large, dirty corneal ulceration with an overhung edge, of chronic duration. Patches of granulation on the lower lid followed by scarring have been reported. Conjunctivitis of different types, pseudomembranous, follicular, or nodular, may develop. Neonatal ophthalmia has been observed. Recently, there have been reports of several cases of intraocular nocardiosis, unknown before except for a single case of postoperative intraocular infection reported by Montarnal in 1965 (François). Chorio-retinitis, postcataract extraction endophthalmitis, and metastatic chorioretinal abscess followed immunosuppressive medication after renal transplant (Jampol et al; Meyer et al; Burpee and Starke).

Treatment. *Nocardia* is sensitive to sulfonamides and to penicillin and other antibiotics.

LEPTOTHRIX

According to the 8th edition of *Bergey's Manual, Leptothrix* is the name applied to the sheathed bacteria commonly found in ponds. These are nonbranching, filamentous bacteria, nonpathogenic, and unrelated to the genus *Actinomyces.*

However, in ophthalmology, *Leptothrix* is of special interest as a cause of conjunctivoglandular Parinaud's syndrome. The condition was first described by Verhoeff in 1918. Using a special staining technique, he demonstrated the organisms in a section of involved tissue. Later, the organism was cultured by Wright, Ridley and Smith, and Gifford and Alexander, either from biopsy or from the pus of the regional glands. The organisms have usually been considered a species of the genus *Actinomyces.* The name is confusing, and more study is needed for identification.

MORPHOLOGY. *Leptothrix* is described in ophthalmology as morphologically similar to *Streptothrix,* except that it is usually unbranched (Plate 30, Fig. 5). To demonstrate *Leptothrix* in section is not easy, and the material has to be obtained from essential lesions. Some filaments are gram-positive, others are gram-negative.

Cultivation is difficult and is seldom done. Positive cultivation on serum-glucose medium and on Brewer's medium has been recorded.

FINDINGS IN THE EYE. Leptothricosis of the eye is rare and is almost exclusively found in children and young adults, chiefly males. The disease appears more commonly in winter. Rabbits, horses, and particularly cats may act as reservoirs for this organism.

The conjunctiva is the only known site of invasion (Kant, Ridley), usually preceded by trauma. The incubation period is three to seven days. Leptothricosis of the conjunctiva is characterized by nodules, single or, more frequently, multiple. They are sometimes pinpoint and scattered on the palpebral conjunctiva and are grayish or yellowish in color. Large, mushroom-shaped lesions may occur. Follicles are usually present. The lids are usually markedly swollen, and enlargement of the preauricular and submaxillary glands (oculoglandular Parinaud's syndrome) is constantly associated with the conditions above.

The bulbar conjunctiva, near the limbus, is most often affected.

The lesions have no tendency to ulcerate, and the cornea is uninvolved.

Catarrhal conjunctivitis of the angular or membranous types may also occur.

TREATMENT.   Iodide or sulfonamides are used systemically. Complete incision of the involved area is indicated. However, even after surgery, the conjunctivitis, as well as enlargement of the preauricular glands, may persist for a long time.

DEEP MYCOSES

Unlike the superficial mycoses, which are usually localized, the deep ones may become systemic or even fatal. Yeastlike fungi are responsible for most of the deep mycoses.

Candida

Many synonyms exist for this large genus, among which *Monilia* was the most popular. Now the name *Candida,* proposed by Berkhout, is generally accepted. *Candida albicans,* among others, is thought to be mostly a pathogenic strain. This is a yeastlike fungus which grows best in environments with a high sugar content, especially fruits. Growth is poor in soil. The fungus has been demonstrated in the normal human flora on mucous membranes of the eye and in the respiratory, gastrointestinal, and female genital tracts. It has also been identified as part of the normal flora in a variety of animals.

The disease, candidiasis, is most common among dishwashers, whose hands remain moist, and among fruit packers.

Overuse of antibiotics and steroids, with consequent disturbance of the normal flora, is believed responsible for the recent increased incidence of candidiasis. The tetracyclines may even stimulate the growth of *Candida.* Pregnancy, alcoholism, vascular stress, and heavy sweating are predisposing factors, as are diabetes, immunosuppressive therapy, and drug addiction.

Morphology. *C. albicans* sometimes has a pseudomycelium yeast morphology, showing a small, ovoid, or cylindric cell four or five times as large as that of staphylococci. The larger size of the individual cells, their budding, and more dense gram-positive staining are important practical criteria in distinguishing *Candida* cells from cocci in the smear. Many of the cells have heavy cell walls which may be composed of cellulose. The cells are most often arranged in irregular, clusterlike masses (Plate 32, Fig. 1). Atypical chains or filaments resembling mycelia are sometimes seen.

Culture. *Candida* species grow on all ordinary media both at room temperature and at 37 C. The use of Sabouraud's glucose agar is preferable, as growth is faster, requiring only three to five days. Blood agar may be used. The colonies are typically cream-colored, small, round, opaque, dry or moist, and resemble staphylococcal colonies (Plate 32, Fig. 3). They produce pseudomycelia and have a distinct yeastlike odor.

Cornmeal agar is used to stimulate the production of chlamydospores (Plate 32, Fig. 2), characteristic for the pathogenic strain.

Pathogenicity and Pathology. Rabbits are particularly susceptible to *C. albicans* and are used to prove pathogenicity. Intravenous injection of 1 ml of 1 percent saline suspension of *C. albicans* infects rabbits and causes death in four to five days. The kidney abscess is characteristic pathology.

Candidiasis is a localized disease which rarely metastasizes. When it does, it may be fatal. Ocular candidiasis is increasingly reported.

The diseases caused by *C. albicans* are thrushlike infections (Plate 31, Fig. 3). They usually develop in newborn children, infected from a mother having vulvovaginitis. Elderly persons, especially if debilitated, are apt to be affected. In generalized cases, the most usual developments are severe lung infections, meningitis, or endocarditis.

Characteristics of the tissue involved and the degree of hypersensitivity to the fungus are the chief factors determining the pathologic picture. The eczematous process, vesicular or pustulous, is typical for the skin infection. Infected mucous membranes have a pseudomembrane, giving a patchy appearance, and for the inner organs, the granulomatous process is characteristic. The granuloma is similar to tuberculous granuloma, with giant epithelial cells, necrosis, and central abscess formation. The fungi are usually found in this necrotic area.

Findings in the Eye. There is no consistency of nomenclature in clinical reports, and the term "monilia" is still frequently used (Mendelblatt, Sykes). Any structure of the eye and its adnexa may be affected by *Candida,* either primarily or secondarily. Although ocular candidiasis is infrequent and uncommon, it now appears to be increasing.

LID CANDIDIASIS. Lesions of the lid skin are usually associated with generalized candidiasis of the face. These are grayish or reddish, scaly, and definitely marginated. Simultaneously, vesicles, pustules, or scaly, red, sharply marginated lesions are found at the lid margins. Eczematous blepharitis or angular blepharoconjunctivitis has also been observed, possibly of allergic origin. Patchy necrotic blepharitis in infants, associated with generalized candidiasis, has been found.

CONJUNCTIVITIS. A pseudomembranous, diffuse or localized, necrotic conjunctivitis followed by ulceration is found in association with similar manifestations of other mucosa. Follicular conjunctivitis can also be seen. A stringy, mucopurulent discharge is commonly present. Lesions of a granulomatous nature may also occur. Norton described thrush of the conjunctiva appearing as four white patches or scabs, symmetrically placed outside the cornea in the palpebral fissure, which were easily removed. The process was indolent, without reaction of the conjunctiva. The condition may be confused with Bitot's spots, and examination of scrapings is essential.

KERATITIS. The manifestations of *Candida* keratitis are varied (Manchester et al; O'Day et al). Peculiar, round, shallow, indolent, gray, and dry corneal ulcers with undermined edges may develop. Near the limbus, the lesions may resemble fascicular keratitis. Central serpiginous hypopyon ulcer resembling a bacterial ulcer may also be caused by *Candida*. A deep ulcer showing a dry necrotic mass resembling bread crumbs (fluorescein stain is often negative), with a pink, glistening base, may occur and may result in perforation and panophthalmitis. This is easily mistaken for a tuberculous infection. A type of dendritic keratitis associated with a foreign body was reported by Sykes. The ulcer was covered by a gray adherent membrane in which *Candida* was revealed.

We have observed two cases of keratitis caused by *C. albicans*. One occurred in generalized candidiasis. Several yellowish infiltrates, sharply marginated, were present. There were also a few small ulcers, covered by masses resembling bread crumbs (Plate 31, Fig. 1). Fluorescein staining was negative. Numerous yeastlike bodies and filamentous forms were found in direct scrapings (Plate 31, Fig. 4). *C. albicans* was identified by cultures, and pathogenicity was proven by injection into a rabbit. The second patient developed a hypopyon ulcerative keratitis after prolonged use of antibiotics. The process was abcesslike and did not respond to treatment (Plate 31, Fig. 2). Several reports have appeared recently regarding endophthalmitis postoperatively or of endogenous origin as caused by *Candida* (Bonatti et al; Michelson et al; Rosen et al). It is characterized by fluffy, white exudates in the posterior vitreous and can be associated with necrotic retinal lesions (Plate 31, Fig. 5). In a comprehensive histopathologic report, Griffin et al and Naumann et al found 6 clinical and 16 postmortem cases showing focal or chorioretinal lesions followed by generalized candidemia.

Infection of the orbit, uveitis, septic retinitis (van Buren), or dacryocystitis (Fine et al; Newton et al) may occasionally develop by continuation from adjacent tissue.

Diagnosis. *C. albicans* is often found in man, either in normal flora or as a secondary invader. Hence it is difficult to prove *Candida* as a primary etiologic agent. Direct examination of fresh material from the lesion is the most important test for diagnosis. One drop of 10 percent potassium hydroxide is added to the exudate, which is then examined in fresh preparation after gentle heating of the slide to clear the exudate.

Staining of the scraping by the gram and Giemsa stains is valuable. Culture and demonstration of chlamydospores are diagnostically important. To demonstrate chlamydospores, direct examination of fresh culture on cornmeal agar is used. Place the plate on the stage, cover the peripheral zone of the growth with a coverglass, and examine under the low-power objective. The chlamydospores appear as thick-walled, terminal cells, being the resting spores of pseudohyphae (Plate 32, Fig. 2).

Skin testing may have value for diagnosis, and it is used to determine and evaluate possible hypersensitivity to the fungus.

There are two distinct antigenic groups: (1) identical with *Candida tropicalis* and (2) identical with *Candida stellatoidea*. The agglutination test or the germ tube test (Plate 32, Fig. 4) is used for identification.

Treatment. Patients with systemic candidiasis or those with hypersensitivity to this fungus present a difficult therapeutic problem.

The localized process may be treated surgically and topically with good results. For topical treatment, any alkaline lotion for the eye may be used. When the disease is external, gentian violet (1 percent solution in 70 percent alcohol) is recommended for painting the skin, including the lid margins. Cauterization of the cornea with tincture of iodine is sometimes effective. In addition, potassium iodide may be given by mouth, provided a skin test is negative for *Candida* hypersensitivity. In hypersensitive patients, potassium iodide may cause dissemination of the disease process. The iodide is usually given by the slow method: starting with 3 drops three times a day, 1 drop is added daily to each dose until 20 drops per dose is reached. The treatment is discontinued in reverse fashion.

Treatment has to be stopped if iodism develops. A low carbohydrate diet is recommended. X-ray therapy may be useful.

Nystatin (Mycostatin) and Mysteclin are usually combined with any of the above-mentioned regimens. Amphotericin B and pimaricin are the preferred drugs (Allen; Berson et al; Bonatti et al; Forster and Rebell; O'Day et al; Rosen et al). Smolin and Okumoto have used antilymphatic serum and corticosteroids.

Blastomyces dermatitidis

Blastomycosis is clinically manifested in three forms: cutaneous, pulmonary, or systemic. The process is usually granulomatous, similar clinically and histologically to tuberculosis. The name "North American blastomycosis" is used. It is also known as "Gilchrist's disease," after the investigator who first described the fungus, *Blastomyces dermatitidis*, in 1896.

Morphology.   The fungus appears in tissue or exudate as a large, spherical, thick-walled, double-contoured, budding, yeastlike body. The organism is smaller in tissue, and may be mistaken for *Histoplasma capsulatum*. On the culture medium, the fungus first appears in the form of yeastlike bodies, which soon become moldlike filaments.

Culture.   The fungus grows readily on Sabourand's medium at room temperature. At first, the colonies are smooth and yeastlike, resembling staphylococci, but hyphal aerial projections quickly develop. The colonies are initially white and cottony (Plate 33, Fig. 2), but later become brownish and prickly. In smear from the colonies, filamentous forms predominate. The filaments, when subcultured, again become yeastlike bodies.

The fungus also grows on blood agar, but more slowly, developing wrinkled, waxy colonies. In smear, budding cells predominate.

Pathology.   Blastomycosis of the skin is a chronic disease which, if untreated, may last for years. The lesions are either papulopustulous or granulomatous and usually result in regional adenopathy. The granuloma frequently turns into an abscess, which is typically surrounded by disseminated, tiny abscesses. The papulopustular lesions generally become ulcerated. Their base is papillary or verrucose and is covered by a dirty pink exudate. The papillary hypertrophy may resemble carcinoma.

The process may become generalized by metastasis to the eye, the lungs or other internal organs, or the bones. The systemic disease is very serious, sometimes fatal.

Findings in the Eye.   Blastomycosis of the eye is relatively uncommon. It has a predilection for the lids (Wilder), appearing in the form of small abscesses around the lashes. According to Wood, the lids may be involved in one-fourth of all cases. The process is destructive and is followed by ectropion and scarring. Blastomycosis of the conjunctiva or cornea is usually secondary to blepharitis. Spreading of the mycosis from the lid margin over the entire face in unrecognized cases has been reported. An opinion exists that the conjunctiva is immune to *B. dermatitidis*, since the process may spread from the lid directly to the cornea, avoiding the conjunctiva. However, blastomycosis of the conjunctiva has been diagnosed by Theodorides and Koutrolikos. The conjunctivitis was characterized by small, whitish spots (resembling Bitot's spots) on the bulbar conjunctiva of the open area. In this case, the identification of blastomycosis cannot be regarded as fully confirmed, since the culture was negative and the diagnosis was made in smear only.

The keratitis (Rodrigues et al; McKee) is rare and usually ulcerative, similar to *Candida* ulcers. Blockage of the nasolacrimal duct by a mycotic mass, resulting in the development of diverticular dacryocystitis, may occur.

Metastatic uveitis in systemic blastomycosis is not as rare as has generally been supposed (Cassady). Metastatic retinal or optic nerve mycoses are unusual manifestations that have been described. Papilledema (Plate 33, Fig. 1) associated with systemic blastomycosis may occur (Schwartz).

Diagnosis. The roof of the lesion must be removed to obtain pus for examination, and the fresh untreated material examined directly. This is mounted on a slide in a drop of 10 percent potassium hydroxide, a coverglass is added, and the slide is gently heated to clear the specimen. The preparation is then examined under subdued light. The thick walls of the budding bodies have a double-contoured appearance characteristic of blastomyces (Plate 33, Fig. 3).

The blastomycin skin test may be valuable, though it can sometimes be positive in healthy persons.

Treatment. If the process is local, excision of the lesion should be performed. Radiation therapy may be useful early in the infection.

The treatment of generalized blastomycosis is a much more difficult problem. Iodides, radiation, or desensitization may be employed. Vaccination is valuable when hypersensitivity exists. Before vaccination, preliminary testing by intracutaneous injection in a dose of 0.1 ml should be performed, then the vaccine diluted according to the size of the skin reaction. Vaccination is highly recommended before starting the iodine treatment, since dissemination of the mycosis may follow iodine therapy.

Stilbamidine or Propamidine may be successfully used. Amphotericin intravenously can be effective.

Histoplasma capsulatum

There are two varieties of histoplasmosis: African, caused by *Histoplasma duboisii* (identified by Dubois in 1952) (Plate 33, Fig. 8), and American, caused by *Histoplasma capsulatum.*

The African type involves the skin, glands, and bones, and organisms are found within giant cells. Ocular involvement is rare but palpebroorbital lesions, lesions of the orbital bones associated with lacrimal glands and conjunctival lesions, can be seen.

American histoplasmosis in the majority of cases is asymptomatic and can only be detected by x-ray examination. The symptomatic form can be either acute or chronic. In the acute, it is usually generalized and the entire reticuloendothelial system can be involved. It can be fatal. In the majority of cases it is initially a lung, oral, or laryngeal infection particularly affecting the tongue (pseudotuberculosis).

H. capsulatum is a yeastlike fungus causing histoplasmosis with varied clinical manifestations. A pure culture of the fungus was obtained in 1934 by De Monbreun. It is a highly infectious mycosis usually appearing as a primary pulmonary disease. Its intracellular nature in the reticuloendothelial system and healing by calcification are characteristics similar to those of *Toxoplasma* infection.

Meleney, reviewing the literature in 1940, found 32 cases of histoplasmosis, with no ocular involvement reported. However, the incidence varies geographically. It is endemic in the Central Mississippi and Ohio valleys, in Oklahoma, and other localities. Incidence is low in Europe and Central America but high in Mexico and Panama.

H. capsulatum may infect many animals, dogs, cats, rodents, or others. The infection is transmitted through biting insects or by animals.

Morphology. *H. capsulatum* is a budding, oval, yeastlike organism usually found within endothelial, mononuclear, or polymorphonuclear cells. The intracellular organisms appear as small, oval bodies resembling protozoa (Plate 33, Fig. 5). The fungus can be demonstrated in exudate, blood smear, or tissue section, stained with Giemsa or Wright stain, and examined with the oil immersion objective. Typical yeastlike budding bodies or tuberculate spores (with projections) are found in fresh preparation from the culture.

Culture. *H. capsulatum* can be cultured on all common laboratory media, at room temperature or at 37 C. On Sabouraud's medium, it grows at room temperature, taking about one month. Initially the growth is cottony and white, becoming brown in older culture (Plate 33, Fig. 6). On blood agar, the growth resembles staphylococci, but a mycelial growth may also occur (Plate 33, Fig. 7).

Pathology. Histoplasmosis is most often found as a primary pulmonary infection, which heals by multiple areas of calcification. It may frequently be manifested as an ulceration of the nasopharyngeal cavities or of the intestine. Generalized adenopathy and secondary anemia or leukopenia usually accompanies the process. Laboratory personnel working with the fungus have been infected. The disease is often asymptomatic, and the patient develops sensitivity to histoplasmin about one week after the initial infection.

Findings in the Eye. Histoplasmosis of the eye is increasingly reported (Olurin et al; Woods et al). The majority of patients showed either peripheral or central chorioretinitis. In 1964 Maumenee reported 61 cases of chorioretinitis. It is already known that histologic investigation showed histoplasmosis in chorioretinitis. A case with a tumorlike ulceration of the palpebral conjunctiva has been recorded (Bruder et al).

Diagnosis.   Determination of the diagnosis is based on finding intracellular yeastlike fungi in peripheral blood smears or other specimens. However, the culture is more important for diagnosis by typical colonies and particularly by tuberculate spores characteristic of *H. capsulatum*. This is demonstrated in wet preparation mounted in cotton blue solution. The typical, spherical, thick-walled spores have finger-like projections (Plate 33, Fig. 4). Chorioretinitis diagnosed by fluorescein technique has been achieved experimentally (Rheins et al). Skin tests can be helpful.

Treatment.   Surgical treatment is indicated for localized histoplasmosis. The generalized process presents a problem, as there is no specific treatment. Iodides, heavy metals, penicillin, or streptomycin may be useful. Amphotericin B intravenously is indicated in severe cases. In most benign cases oral sulfa drugs can be effective.

Cryptococcus neoformans

Cryptococcus is a yeastlike fungus, nonsporulating and nonmycelial. The species *Cryptococcus neoformans* is pathogenic for man. Soil, milk, and especially pigeons' nests are considered the most common sources of infection.

C. neoformans may involve any part of the body but has a predilection for the central nervous system. Chronic meningitis is a typical manifestation of cryptococcosis, and the ocular nervous tissue is often secondarily involved.

Morphology.   Cryptococci are large, thick-walled, budding bodies, round or elongated. These are usually arranged in a honeycomb-appearing mass (Plate 34, Fig. 6). The organism is surrounded by a thick, gelatinous capsule, usually twice as wide as the cell body. The capsule is best demonstrated with India ink, in fresh preparation (Plate 34, Fig. 3).

Culture.   The fungus grows on Sabouraud's medium, slowly and at room temperature. Colonies appear white, wrinkled, and granular. Later, they become moist and shiny, have a tendency to coalesce, and are tan to brown in color (Plate 34, Fig. 7). Budding cells are found, and a capsule is readily demonstrated at this stage. There is no spore formation. On blood agar, the colonies are gray, opaque, round, and glistening, resembling staphylococci.

Pathology.   Primary lesions are mainly found in the lungs, rarely on the skin or mucosa, and are associated with adenopathy. The organisms may spread to the brain, causing chronic meningitis lasting many years and resembling a brain tumor. The signs are the same as in any other meningitis, but despite the severity of the symptoms, acute inflammation is usually absent.

Human transmission of the mycosis is unknown.

Findings in the Eye.   The eye is rarely involved, usually secondarily to meningitis. Ocular symptoms of the meningitis are amblyopia, strabismus, nystagmus, ptosis, and diplopia. Neuroretinitis (Plate 34, Fig. 2), choked disk, and cystoid degeneration or hemorrhages of the retina have been observed. A case of intraocular cryptococcosis has been described by Weiss et al. This appeared as a binocular cystic growth in the retina, from which *C. neoformans* was isolated. Orbital cryptococcosis has been reported. The fungus has also been found by Cohen in association with Hodgkin's disease. The eyebrow can be the site of a primary lesion (Plate 34, Fig. 1). Many cases of metastatic chorioretinitis and detachment of the retina have been reported in both adults and children (Khodadoust et al; Okun et al). Endophthalmitis in cases of meningitis can occur, and spontaneous regression is known.

Diagnosis of cryptococcic mycosis is difficult for the ophthalmologist and is usually made postmortem. (For exception, see Weiss et al.)

Diagnosis.   This is determined by finding *C. neoformans* either in the specimen or in the culture. The material may be obtained by aspiration, swabbing, or scraping the tissue from the biopsy specimen. Mount the material in a drop of diluted India ink and examine it under a coverglass while the preparation is wet (Plate 34, Fig. 3); avoid drying. India ink is used for contrast with the capsule. The wide capsule is important for differential diagnosis (Plate 34, Figs. 3, 4). The frozen section of tissue is mounted in undiluted Giemsa stain. The periodic acid–Schiff (PAS) technique also gives an excellent result. The fungus in section is found free or within giant cells. To prove the pathogenicity of the organisms, a cultural suspension is injected into mice intraperitoneally, intracerebrally, or intravenously.

Virulence of the strain is indicated by meningitis or death of the mice.

Treatment.   Actidione and amphotericin B have been recommended. Intravenous amphotericin B (30 mg daily) is effective in the disseminated process. Good results have been recorded with intravenous Mycostatin. The addition of sulfonamides to the above treatments may be helpful.

PITYROSPORUM OVALE AND *PITYROSPORUM ORBICULARIS*

Pityrosporum ovale (PO) is of particular interest to the ophthalmologist. While it is an almost constant finding in seborrhea, opinions as to its etiologic role are varied. Whether or not *P. ovale* is a cause of seborrhea, its presence is of diagnostic value.

Pityrosporum orbicularis was first discovered by Gordon in 1951. There is little difference between *P. orbicularis* and *P. ovale* except that *P. orbicularis* is more fastidious in its growth requirements, and morphologically, it is round, whereas *P. ovale* is oval. *P. orbicularis* is commonly found on the lid margins (Parunovic and Halde).

The yeastlike fungus does not produce a mycelium. Because of its lipolytic properties, the organism does not fit into any group.

Morphology. The typical yeastlike budding bodies vary in form, being either spherical, ovoid, cylindrical, or flask-shaped. Round forms may predominate over the oval in the scrapings from the lid margin (Plate 36, Figs. 2, 3) and in the acute process. Flask-shaped forms are more common in dandruff. They are gram-positive and usually stain deeply. Staining with methylene blue is preferable. The slide must be heat-fixed and stained with methylene blue for five minutes. It should be washed carefully during staining, as the greasy specimen may slide off.

The organism is distinguished from staphylococci by its large size, budding forms, and dense gram staining.

Culture. Cultivation of *P. ovale* is extremely difficult because of its lipolytic properties. A great achievement in cultivation was made by Benham (1941). It was shown that wort agar, containing oleic acid, and Littman's agar, with olive oil, are the most suitable media. Growth is more successful on Littman's agar (Plate 36, Fig. 4). The colonies resemble staphylococcal colonies. They have a greasy appearance and may float on the oil. A cheesy odor is characteristic. Cultivation is still difficult and often negative. Growth takes about seven days, contaminating molds are not uncommon, and staphylococci or other bacteria are invariably present. Subculture requires about two to five days, and growth can be achieved on Sabouraud's medium (Plate 36, Fig. 5) or blood agar if oil is added. Giant colonies may develop.

Dandruff or seborrheic scales are used as specimens. As many scales as possible should be scraped from the lid margin, seeded on the plate, then immediately covered with olive oil in a thick layer, sealed, and incubated at 37 C. The growth must be checked frequently.

Seborrhea and P. ovale. Hypersecretion of the sebaceous glands, including the meibomian glands, is the basis for seborrhea. This lipid secretion is favorable for the growth of *P. ovale*. Although not a cause of seborrhea, the organism may play an important role in its development, either aggravating the process or causing a sensitization of the involved tissue. A number of factors are important in the pathogenesis of seborrhea: systemic disturbances, chiefly of the endocrine system, or constipation, indigestion, excessive use of alcohol or tobacco, some chronic diseases, particularly tuberculosis or syphilis, or familial tendency.

Findings in the Eye. Thygeson was the first to make a thorough study of the relationship of *P. ovale* and seborrheic blepharitis. The evidence concerning its etiologic role was inconclusive. However, he showed a definite relationship between the number of organisms present and the severity of the process.

Seborrheic blepharitis, the basis of which is hypersecretion of the meibomian glands, is the most common type. It is almost always part of a general seborrheic state and is usually associated with dandruff. The condition is characterized by greasy scales (Plate 36, Fig. 1). Persons of dark complexion have an extensive hypersecretion, and the scales are thick and greasy. The hypersecretion is less in blonds, and the scales are drier. Blepharitis is chronic, lasting for years, with recurrent attacks and is very stubborn to treat. The eyes are very sensitive to irritants (eg, light, heat, cold, smoke). This can be an asymptomatic condition, but its effects cannot be ignored. The meibomian orifices may be dilated or obstructed or covered by an epithelial oil-retaining cyst situated along the inner edge of the lid margin. These cysts are easily ruptured, and the oil drains, leaving a small crater. This is important diagnostically and was described by Keith (London). The secretion is usually fluid, transparent or turbid. Recently many other conditions associated with blepharitis have been described. In the majority of cases papillae are present, also follicles for which a viral etiology could be wrongly suspected. Corneal involvement can be associated with seborrheic blepharitis more often than is suggested, eg, superficial punctate keratitis (SPK), diffuse epithelial keratitis (possibly can be confused with herpes), pannus formation, and keratoconjunctivitis sicca. Episcleritis has also been seen.

The condition is often aggravated by secondary bacterial infection, especially *Staphylococcus aureus.* Then the inflammation becomes more severe, the lid margins ulcerate and thicken, and sties and chalazia frequently occur. Seborrheic blepharitis is chronic and may last for years or for an entire lifetime. Periodic exacerbations are typical. Hair follicles may atrophy as a result of such a prolonged process, and madarosis may follow. A chronic conjunctivitis usually accompanies the blepharitis. Marginal corneal ulcers are not uncommon.

Treatment. There is no really effective treatment. Local therapy should be combined with general treatment of the seborrheic state, especially the dandruff.

Lid hygiene is of the utmost importance. Swabbing of the above-mentioned epithelial cyst and cleaning the lid margins with alkaline lotion are suggested before any other local treatment. Twice daily applications of ointment, 1 percent ammoniated mercury and 1 percent salicylic acid in petrolatum, may give a good result (Thygsen). Painting of the lid margins with 2 percent silver nitrate can be used. Expression of secretion from the meibomian glands, followed by massage, is highly recommended. For bacterial infection, suitable antibiotics should be given, although it is important to avoid overtreatment.

Limiting carbohydrate intake in the diet is also important.

ASPERGILLUS

Aspergillus is a large genus of fungi widely distributed in soil, water, air, and animal products. They are the most common and troublesome laboratory contaminants, being frequently found on Sabouraud's medium. Among the many species, *Aspergillus fumigatus* is most often associated with infection, either as a secondary invader or as a primary cause of disease. Aspergillosis is frequent in plants, insects, birds, particularly penguins, animals, both wild and domestic, and man. Sometimes it causes great economic loss. The incidence in man is greater in adult males and among workers in an environment contaminated by spores, eg, squab raisers, furriers using rye flour as a grease remover, or farmers. The increase in aspergillosis is associated with the immunosuppressive state, leukemia, and lymphoma, with the prolonged use of antibiotics, and especially with corticosteroids.

Morphology. *A. fumigatus* or *Aspergillus niger* may appear in exudate or other specimens as broken fragments of hyphae, together with numerous round, dark green or black, scattered spores. Culture is needed for identification.

Culture. The fungus is fast-growing at room temperature, with white, filamentous, cottony colonies which become velvety. Later, the colonies are green or dark green in *A. fumigatus*, characteristic for spore production. In *A. niger* the colonies are black and powdery (Plate 37, Fig. 3).

Diagnosis. Whether *Aspergillus* is a secondary invader or a primary cause of disease is difficult to determine. The presence of spores and their typical arrangements are diagnostically important. They are demonstrated best in wet preparation of the specimen or in direct examination of the colony. The tube is placed on the stage, and the edge of the colony is studied under the low-power objective. The conidiophore which is characteristic of *Aspergillus* is terminated by a vesicle covered with sterigmata. The latter have long chains of spores. In wet preparation, which is essential, hyphae with characteristic heads are apparent, and these are diagnostic (Plate 37, Fig. 4).

Pathology.   The ear is the most common site of infection, which is also found in the orbit and eye, the sinuses, lungs, bronchi, and skin. Aspergillosis is usually a chronic granulomatous process which can be disseminated and is often fatal (Green et al; Lederman and Madge). However, the pathology differs according to the tissue involved. The process in the sinuses and eye is usually pyogenic, resembling a bacterial process but distinguished by the periodic appearance of greenish masses containing the fungus. Infection of the nails simulates those of dermatophytes. A mass of the fungus may be found within cavities, a so-called aspergilloma, which can cause obstruction.

Findings in the Eye.   Occurrences of ocular aspergillosis have been increasingly reported, and some have been severe, resulting in loss of the globe, eg, in a drug addict (Getnick et al). Aspergillosis of the orbit (Green et al), probably a continuation from the sinuses, is known. Fumigatus corneal ulcer, followed by perforation and loss of the globe, has been described by Castroveijo and Muñoz Urra. Intraocular posttraumatic aspergillosis, including postoperative, has been reported (Darrel; Rychener). Aspergillosis of the orbit, blepharitis, or dacryocystitis may occur. The incidence of fungal ocular infections is probably much greater than has been diagnosed. Therefore, Birge in reviewing mycotic diseases of the eye, has emphasized that the so-called saprophytic fungi must be reevaluated.

Treatment.   Surgical treatment followed by iodides is usually indicated for localized granuloma, and drainage is suggested for abscesses. In processes that cannot be treated surgically, slow or rapid iodide therapy was formerly used. However, amphotericin B is the drug of choice (Harrell et al).

MUCOR

The mucor fungi (phycomycetes), like aspergilli, are constant contaminants in cultures of clinical material. They are widely distributed in soil, manure, and fruits, being commonly known as bread molds. However, the *Mucor* genus is extremely pathogenic for man, causing mucormycosis in patients with uncontrolled diabetes mellitus. Mucormycosis has been most often described in Germany. It is not transmitted from man to man.

Morphology.   The fungus can be readily demonstrated in periodic acid-Schiff (PAS), hematoxylin-eosin, and silver preparations, as large, broad, nonseptate, branching hyphae.

Culture.   The fungus grows quickly on Sabouraud's medium and fills the test tube or petri dish with large grayish mycelia in three to four days. Detailed cultural studies are required, since these fungi in cases of mucormycosis have mostly been described postmortem.

Pathology. Mucormycosis is rapidly fatal, within one to five days. The infection mainly affects the brain or lungs. However, the brain can be secondarily involved by initial invasion of the orbit or sinuses. The process is usually characterized by acute inflammation and by vascular thrombi in which the fungus has been revealed.

Findings in the Eye. Acute orbital cellulitis is the most common ocular manifestation of mucormycosis (Gass). The process is usually continued from sinusitis and spreads to the brain, causing meningoencephalitis. The associated symptoms are proptosis, internal hemoplegia, and external hemoplegia. Only three cases of chronic ocular manifestation are known. Two of them are keratomycoses, and one an intraocular mycosis resembling Coats' disease, described by Wadsworth, which was not associated with diabetes.

Treatment. In any suspected case, treatment should be started at once. This includes use of systemic antifungal drugs, such as intravenous amphotericin B, oral nystatin (Mycostatin), or potassium iodide. Antibiotics are administered for secondary bacterial infections.

SUPERFICIAL MYCOSES

This section is concerned with superficial fungal infections of the skin and its derivatives, such as hair and nails. Systemic involvement is almost unknown. Dermatomycosis is widely distributed, although it has some geographic preference. It is estimated that one-half of the population of the United States sooner or later develops this disease.

Fungal species causing the dermatomycoses are divided into three genera: *Trichophyton, Epidermophyton,* and *Microsporum.*

Numerous names are confusingly applied either to the fungi or to the mycoses: their complicated classifications are matters for the mycologist.

The superficial mycoses are rare in ophthalmology. A few comments pertinent to ophthalmology will be given.

Morphology. This varies in different species. The fungus appears as mycelial fragments or long, branching filaments (from the culture). Mycelia may break up into arthrospores, which are spores formed by fragmentation of hyphae. They are arranged in various patterns, such as mosaics, sheaths, or parallel rows, in different species. The study of spores is most important for the individual diagnosis of dermatomycosis.

For microscopic examination, place the infectious material on a slide (with a drop of 10 percent to 40 percent potassium hydroxide, depending on species), heat gently to clear material, and examine under a coverglass. Direct microscopic examination is very valuable for the diagnosis. Specific identification can only be done by cultivation.

Cultivation.   Cultivation is on Sabouraud's medium at room temperature, growth taking two to three weeks. The colonies are powdery, cottony, or velvety, and of varying colors—pink, red, white, or brownish.

Pathology.   The fungus infects only superficial keratinized epithelial tissue and grows so superficially that it resembles colony formation on the surface of a medium. The tissue reaction is very mild: light redness, edema, scaling, vesicle formation, and thickening of the keratinized layer may occur. Secondary infection is common. Then the process becomes more severe, resembling pyogenic infection, and the regional lymph glands may be enlarged. Tinea is characterized by spread of the fungus circularly from the center. Healing from the inside out, it leaves characteristic rings.

Hypersensitivity to fungal products may frequently develop elsewhere on the body, especially the hands, and usually results in the formation of vesicles.

Though dermatomycosis is a superficial process, it may be very troublesome, as it is chronic and often incurable. The fungi are chiefly transmitted from cats or dogs to children. The infections are more severe in tropical countries.

Clinical Features.   The most common type of dermatomycosis is tinea, or ringworm, having ring-shaped lesions. Tinea may occur in various parts of the body. There are distinguished tinea capitis, tinea barbae or sycosis, and tinea pedis or athlete's foot. The fungus *Microsporum audouinii* is commonly found in both man and domestic animals. Any part of the body may be infected. In children, the scalp is especially sensitive, while the feet are resistant, and the opposite is true in adults.

Findings in the Eye.   Tinea circinata of the lid skin occurs very rarely and is usually secondary to involvement of the face or scalp. Trichophytosis of the lid may show a very slight inflammation which is patchy in appearance; sometimes a purulent ulcer occurs. The mycosis of the lid margin is scaly or purulent, the latter generally caused by a superimposed bacterial infection.

The regional lymph glands may be enlarged. The cilia or the hairs of the eyebrow are often lost as a result of folliculitis of the hair.

Treatment.   The infected epithelial structure should be removed and the infected hair epilated. Application of tincture of iodine or ointments, such as salicylic acid, ammoniated mercury, or sodium propionate, has been used effectively. A compress with potassium permanganate solution is recommended.

REFERENCES

Fungi

Aldridge JS, Kirk R: Mycetoma of the eyelid. Br J Ophthalmol 24:211, 1940

Anderson B, Roberts SS Jr, Gonzalez C, Chick EW: Mycotic ulcerative keratitis. Arch Ophthalmol 62:169, 1959

Ashine JW, Ellis PP: Endophthalmitis and contact lenses. Am J Ophthalmol 66:960, 1968

Birge HL: Ocular aspects of mycotic infection. Arch Ophthalmol 47:354, 1952

Brown SI, Bloomfield S, Pearce D et al: Infections with the therapeutic soft lens. Arch Ophthalmol 91:275, 1974

Buchanan RE, Gibbons NE (eds): Bergey's Manual of Determinative Bacteriology, 8th ed. Baltimore, Williams & Wilkins, 1974

Fazakas S: Comprehensive report on secondary mycoses in diseases of the palpebral margin, the conjunctiva and the cornea. Surv Ophthalmol 5:419, 1960

Francois J: Oculomycosis. Springfield, Ill., Charles C. Thomas, 1972

Hammeke JC, Ellis PP: Mycotic flora of the conjunctiva. Am J Ophthalmol 49:1174, 1960

Henly W, Okas S, Waithe W et al: Cellular immunity in chronic disorders (lymphocytes stimulation and protein synthesis). Am J Ophthalmol 73:56, 1972

Joklik WK, Smith DT: Zinsser Microbiology, 16th ed. New York, Appleton, 1976

Jones B: Principal in the management of oculomycosis XXXI: Edward Jackson Memorial Lecture. Am J Ophthalmol 79:719, 1975

Kaufman HE, Wood RM: Mycotic keratitis. Am J Ophthalmol 59:993, 1965

Levitt JM: Ocular manifestations of coccidioidomycosis. Am J Ophthalmol 31:1626, 1948

Ley AP, Sanders TE: Fungus keratitis. Arch Ophthalmol 56:257, 1956

Mitsui Y, Hanabusa J: Corneal infections after cortisone therapy. Br J Ophthalmol 39:244, 1955

Naumann G, Green WR, Zimmerman LE: Mycotic keratitis. Am J Ophthalmol 64:668, 1967

Olson CL: Fungal contamination of the conjunctiva and lid margin. Arch Ophthalmol 81:351, 1969

Palmer E, Ferry A, Safir A: Fungal invasion of a soft (Griffin biomite) contact lens. Arch Ophthalmol 93:278, 1975

Polack FM, Kaufman HE, Newmark E: Keratomycosis: medical and surgical treatment. Arch Ophthalmol 85:410, 1971

Rychener RO: Intra-ocular mycosis. Trans Am Ophthalmol Soc 31:4, 1933

Simon FA: Allergic conjunctivitis due to fungi. JAMA 110:440, 1938

Smolin G, Okumoto M: Antilymphocyte serum potentiation of candida keratitis. Am J Ophthalmol 66:804, 1968

Thygeson P, Hogan M, Kimura S: Cortisone and hydrocortisone in ocular infections. Trans Am Acad Ophthal 57:64, 1953

Tomar V, Sharma O, Joski A: Bacterial and fungal flora of normal conjunctiva. Ann Ophthal 3:669, 1971

Wilson LA, Achern D, Jones D, Sexton R: Fungi from the normal outer eye. Am J Ophthalmol 67:52, 1969

Wilson LA, Sexton RR: Laboratory diagnosis in fungal keratitis. Am J Ophthalmol 66:646, 1968

Actinomyces and Leptothrix

Benedict WL, Iverson HA: Chronic keratoconjunctivitis associated with nocardia. Arch Ophthalmol 32:89, 1944

Bruce GM, Locatcher-Khorazo D: Actinomyces: recovery of the streptothrix in a case of superficial punctate keratitis. Arch Ophthalmol 27:294, 1942

Buchanan RE, Gibbons NE (eds): Bergey's Manual of Determinative Bacteriology, 8th ed. Baltimore, Williams & Wilkins, 1974

Burpee JC, Starke WR: Bilateral metastatic intraocular nocardiosis. Arch Ophthalmol 86:666, 1971

Elliot AJ: Streptothricosis of the lacrimal canaliculi. Am J Ophthalmol 24:682, 1941

Ellis PP, Bausor SC, Fulmer JM: Streptothrix canaliculitis. Am J Ophthalmol 52:36, 1961

Gibson JM: Actinomycosis of the canaliculi with invasion of tissue in one case. Br J Ophthalmol 36:522, 1952

Gifford SR, Day AA: Leptotrichosis conjunctivae. Arch Ophthalmol 31:423, 1944

Jampol LM, Strauch B, Albert D: Intraocular nocardiosis. Am J Ophthalmol 76:568, 1973

Kant A: Unusual case of leptothricosis conjunctivae. Am J Ophthalmol 31:607, 1948

Lemoine AN: Parinaud's conjunctivitis, with demonstration of the leptothrix of Verhoeff. JAMA 82:537, 1924

Meyer SL, Fonti R, Shaver R: Intraocular nocardiosis. Arch Ophthalmol 83:536, 1970

Nagel CSG: Fungus concretion in lacrimal canaliculus (streptothricosis, actinomycosis). Am J Ophthalmol 3:327, 1920

Penikett EJK, Rees DL: Nocardia asteroides infection. Am J Ophthalmol 53:1006, 1962

Pine L, Hardin H: Actinomyces israelii: a cause of lacrimal canaliculitis in man. J Bacteriol 78:164, 1959

Pine L, Hardin H, Turner L, Roberts SS: Actinomycotic lacrimal canaliculitis. Am J Ophthalmol 49:1278, 1960

Ridley F, Smith C: Leptotrichosis conjunctivae. Br J Ophthalmol 36:328, 1952

Sanford AH, Voelker M: Actinomycosis in the United States. Arch Surg 11:809, 1925

Schardt WM, Unsworth AC, Hayes CV: Corneal ulcer due to Nocardia asteroides. Am J Ophthalmol 43:303, 1956

Smith CH: Ocular actinomycosis. Proc R Soc Med 46:209, 1953

Theodore FH: Streptothrix as a cause of follicular conjunctivitis and other obscure conjunctivitides. Am J Ophthalmol 33:1225, 1950

Thorson JA, Mueller EF: Probable actinomycosis of the orbit. J Iowa Med Soc 31:70 1941

Verhoeff FH: Observations on Parinaud's conjunctivitis (leptothricosis conjunctivae). Am J Ophthalmol 1:705, 1918

Wright RE: Isolation of Verhoeff's leptothrix in a case of Parinaud's syndrome. Arch Ophthalmol 18:233, 1937

Deep Mycoses

Allen H: Amphotericin B and exogenous mycotic endophthalmitis after cataract extraction. Arch Ophthalmol 88:640, 1972

Beamer PR, Smith EB, Barnett HL: Histoplasmosis: report of case in infant and experimental observations. J Pediatr 24:270, 1944

Berson EL, et al: Treatment of experimental fungal keratitis. Arch Ophthalmol 74:403, 1965

Birge HL: The diagnosis of ocular mycotic infections. Arch Ophthalmol 46:225, 1951

Bonatti WD, Jaeger E, Frayer W: Endogenous fungal endophthalmitis. Arch Ophthalmol 70: 772, 1963

Broders AC, Dochat GR, Herrell WE, Vaughn LD: An unusual case of histoplasmosis. Proc Staff Meet Mayo Clin 19:123, 1944

Cassady JV: Uveal blastomycosis. Arch Ophthalmol 35:84, 1946

Chin GN, Hyndiuk R, Kwasny G, Schultz R: Keratomycosis in Wisconsin. Am J Ophthalmol 79:121, 1975

Cohen M: Binocular papilledema in a case of torulosis associated with Hodgkin's disease. Arch Ophthalmol 32:477, 1944

De Monbreun WA: The cultivation and cultural characteristics of Darling's *Histoplasma capsulatum*. Am J Trop Med Hyg 14:93, 1934

Ferguson AS: Blastomycosis of eye and face secondary to lung infection. Br Med J 1:442, 1928

Fine M, Waring WS: Mycotic obstruction of the nasolacrimal duct (*Candida albicans*). Arch Ophthalmol 38:39, 1947

Forster RK, Rebell G: The diagnosis and management of keratomycosis. Arch Ophthalmol 93:975, 1975

Francois J, Ryseelaere M: Oculmycoses. Springfield, Ill, Thomas, 1972

Griffin JR, Pettit T, Fishman L, Foos R: Blood-borne *Candida* endophthalmitis. A clinical and pathological study of 21 cases. Arch Ophthalmol 89:450, 1973

Hiles DA, Font RL: Bilateral intraocular cryptococcosis; unilateral spontaneous regression. Am J Ophthalmol 65:98, 1968

Kallet HA, McKenzie K, Johnson F: Bacterial pseudomycosis of the orbit. Am J Ophthalmol 68:504, 1969

Khodadoust A, Payne J: Cryptococcal (torular) retinitis. Am J Ophthalmol 67:745, 1969

Krause AC, Hopkins WG: Ocular manifestation of histoplasmosis. Am J Ophthalmol 34:564, 1951

Manchester PT Jr, Georg LK: Corneal ulcer due to *Candida parapsilosis (C. parakrusei)*. JAMA 171:1339, 1959

Maumenee AE: The contribution of immunology to clinical ophthalmology. Am J Ophthalmol 58:230, 1964

McKee SH: Blastomycoses of the cornea. Internat Clin 3:50, 1926

Meleney HE: Histoplasmosis (reticulo-endothelial cytomycosis). Am J Trop Med Hyg 20:603, 1940

Mendelblatt DL: Moniliasis. Am J Ophthalmol 36:379, 1953

Michelson P, Rupp R, Efthimiadis B: Endogenous candida endophthalmitis. Am J Ophthalmol 80:800, 1975

Milausckas AT: Mycotic scleral abscess following a scleral buckling operation. Am J Ophthalmol 63:951, 1967

Mitsui Y, Hanabusa J: Corneal infections after cortisone therapy. Br J Ophthalmol 39:244, 1955

Naumann G, Green G, Zimmerman W: Mycotic keratitis. A histopathological study of 73 cases. Am J Ophthalmol 64:668, 1967

Newton JC, Tulevech CB: Lacrimal canaliculitis due to Candida albicans. Am J Ophthalmol 53:933, 1962

Norton AH: Thrush of the conjunctiva. Am J Ophthalmol 10:357, 1927

O'Day D, Moore T, Aronson S: Deep fungal corneal abscess. Arch Ophthalmol 86:414, 1971

Okun E, Butler W: Ophthalmologic cryptococcal meningitis. Arch Ophthal 71:52, 1964

Olurin O, Lucas A, Oyldiran A: Orbital histoplasmosis due to Histoplasma duboisii. Am J Ophthalmol 68:14, 1969

Rheins MS, Pixley PA, Suie T, et al: Diagnosis of experimental fungal ulcers by fluorescein antibody technique. Am J Ophthalmol 62:892, 1966

Rodrigues MM, Laibson P, Kaplan W: Exogenous mycotic keratitis caused by Blastomyces dermatitidis. Am J Ophthalmol 85:782, 1973

Rosen R, Fridman A: Successfully treated post-operative Candida parakrusei endophthalmitis. Am J Ophthalmol 76:574, 1973

Schwartz VJ: Intra-ocular blastomycosis. Arch Ophthalmol 5:581, 1931

Smolin G, Okumoto M: Potentiation of Candida albicans keratitis by antilymphatic serum and corticosteroids. Am J Ophthalmol 68:675, 1969

Sykes EM: Fungus infection of the cornea: case report of keratomycosis due to Monilia. Tex J Med 42:330, 1946

Theodorides E, Koutrolikos D: Blastomycosis of the conjunctiva. Am J Ophthalmol 36:978, 1953

Van Buren JM: Septic retinitis due to Candida albicans (Abstract). Am J Ophthalmol 46:277, 1958

Weiss C, Perry IH, Shevky MC: Infection of the human eye with Cryptococcus neoformans (Torula histolytica; Cryptococcus hominis). Arch Ophthalmol 39:739, 1948

Wilder WH: Blastomycosis of the eyelid. JAMA 43:2026, 1904

Wood CA: Blastomycosis of the ocular structures, especially of the eyelids. Ann Ophthalmol 13:92, 1904

Woods AC, Wahlen HE: The probable role of benign histoplasmosis in the etiology of granulomatous uveitis. Am J Ophthalmol 49:205, 1960

Pityrosporum ovale, Aspergillus, Mucor, Superficial Mycoses

Andrew PF: Cerebral mucormycosis (phycomycosis): Ocular findings and review of literature. Surv Ophthalmol 6:1, 1961

Baker RD: Mucormycosis—a new disease? JAMA 163:805, 1957

Benham RW: Pityrosporum ovale: a lipophilic fungus. Thiamin and oxaloacetic acid as growth factors. Proc Soc Exp Biol Med 58:199, 1945

Benham RW: Cultural characteristics of Pityrosporum ovale: a lipophilic fungus. Nutrient and growth requirements. Proc Soc Exp Biol Med 46:176, 1941

Benham RW: The cultural characteristics of Pityrosporum ovale: lipophilic fungus. J Invest Dermatol 2:187, 1939

Birge HL: The diagnosis of ocular mycotic infections. Arch Ophthalmol 46:225, 1951

Castroviejo R, Muñoz Urra F: Aspergillosis ocular. Arch Oftalmol Hispano-Am 21:453, 1921

Cogan DG: Endogenous intraocular fungous infection. Arch Ophthalmol 42: 666, 1949

Darrel RW: Endogenous *Aspergillus* uveitis following heart surgery. Arch Ophthalmol 78:354, 1967

Donahue HC: Unusual mycotic infection of the lacrimal canaliculi and conjunctiva. Am J Ophthalmol 32:207, 1949

Emmons CW: The isolation and pathogenicity of P.O.. Weekly Public Health Rep 55 (Part 2):1306, 1940

Gass JDM: Mucormycosis: review. Arch Ophthalmol 65:226, 1961

Getnick R, Rodrigues M: Endogenous fungal endophthalmitis in a drug addict. Am J Ophthalmol 77:680, 1974

Gots JS, Thygeson P, Waisman M: Observations on *Pityrosporum ovale* in seborrheic blepharitis and conjunctivitis. Am J Ophthalmol 65:226, 1961

Green WB, Font RL, Zimmerman LE: Aspergillosis of the orbit. Report of 10 cases and review of the literature. Arch Ophthalmol 82:302, 1969

Harley RD, Mishler JE: Endogenous intraocular fungus infections. Trans Am Acad Ophthalmol 63:264, 1959

Harrell ER, Walter JR, Gutow RF, et al: Localized aspergillosis of the eyelid. Treatment with local amphotericin B. Arch Ophthalmol 76:322, 1966

Keith CG: Seborrheic blepharo-keratoconjunctivitis. Trans Ophthalmol Soc UK 87:85, 1967

Lederman IR, Madge G: Endogenous intraocular aspergillosis. Arch Ophthalmol 76:233, 1966

Parunovic A, Halde C: *Pityrosporum orbiculare.* Am J Ophthalmol 63:815, 1967

Rosenvold LK: Dacryocystitis and blepharitis due to infection by *Aspergillus niger.* Am J Ophthalmol 25:588, 1942

Rychener RO: Intra-ocular mycosis. Trans Am Ophthalmol Soc 31:477, 1933

Stern SG, Kulvin MM: Aspergillosis of the cornea. Am J Ophthalmol 33:111, 1950

Stratemeier WP: Mucormycosis of the central nervous system. Arch Neurol Psychiat 63:179, 1950

Thygeson P: Etiology and treatment of blepharitis. Arch Ophthalmol 36:445, 1946

Veirs ER, Davis CT: Fungus infections of the eye and the orbit. Arch Ophthalmol 59:172, 1958

Vidal F: Zeissitis caused by the round *Pityrosporum* (abstract). Am J Ophthalmol 36:1181, 1953

Vidal F, Weil BA: Sebaceous blepharosis. Am J Ophthalmol 36:421, 1953

Wadsworth JAC: Ocular mucormycosis. Am J Ophthalmol 34:405, 1951

Wright RE: Two cases of granuloma invading the orbit due to an *Aspergillus.* Br J Ophthalmol 11:545, 1927

5

Clinical and Laboratory Techniques in External Ocular Disease and Endophthalmitis

ROBERT A. HYNDIUK
SAM SEIDEMAN

The ophthalmologist can find the laboratory very useful when confronted with an external disease problem in which there is any doubt about the diagnosis. During residency training and in the early days of practice, the ophthalmologist should use the laboratory extensively to correlate etiology and clinical findings. Once comfortable with correlation of laboratory findings and clinical findings, one can usually do without laboratory help except in certain cases where it is necessary to do laboratory studies:

1. Corneal ulcers, where bacterial or fungal infection is suspected
2. Hyperacute conjunctivitis
3. Membranous conjunctivitis
4. Any moderately severe long-standing conjunctivitis
5. Ophthalmia neonatorum
6. Postoperative infections, endophthalmitis
7. Parinaud's ocular glandular syndrome

Supported by a grant from The Hearst Foundations, by Training Grant Account 5T01-EY00045-09 and in part by an unrestricted grant from Research to Prevent Blindness; from the Cornea–External Disease Unit, Department of Ophthalmology, Medical College of Wisconsin, and the Milwaukee County Medical Complex, Milwaukee, Wisconsin.

8. Periocular abscess
9. The overtreated red eye

At other times, one will be presented with external disease problems in which cultures and scrapings, although not absolutely necessary, are often very helpful in arriving at a diagnosis:

1. Allergic conjunctivitis (vernal, atopic)
2. Chronic conjunctivitis
3. Canaliculitis, dacryocystitis
4. Persistent blepharitis unresponsive to therapy
5. Infectious eczematoid conjunctivitis

This chapter will serve as a guide and will include practical and general information on office techniques of obtaining specimens and some general information about ocular microbiology and cytology, to help the ophthalmologist in the clinic or office.

TECHNIQUES OF OBTAINING SPECIMENS

CULTURES

Routine cultures of conjunctiva and lid margins are usually taken on blood agar. However, when a patient has a hyperacute purulent conjunctivitis, one should suspect *Neisseria,* and chocolate agar should be used. Cultivation on chocolate agar should also be included when investigating bacterial conjunctivitis in a young child, especially if it is associated with an orbital cellulitis or otitis media *(Haemophilus* may be involved). Long-standing blepharitis is usually caused by staphylococci, but rarely a fungal infection may be present. Sabouraud's medium is indicated, or a separate blood agar plate may be inoculated and kept at room temperature if a Sabouraud's plate is not immediately available. In the case of a corneal ulcer or endophthalmitis in which one suspects either a bacterial or fungal infection, one should culture directly to blood agar, chocolate agar, Sabouraud's medium, and enriched liquid broth, eg, brain-heart infusion broth or chopped meat broth. Anaerobic cultures need special media, which will be discussed.

Lid and Conjunctival Cultures

Routine conjunctival and lid margin cultures should be taken without topical anesthesia, as anesthetics and their preservatives have some antibacterial properties, especially if they are incorporated in the specimen. Cultures can be taken without discomfort using the following technique. The lower lid is everted, and the entire lower cul-de-sac is wiped, using a sterile cotton-tipped applicator which has been moistened with sterile broth (Plate 45, Fig. 1). The applicator is then used to streak the agar plate directly. Such a moistened swab increases the recovery of organisms over the recovery possible when using dry swabs. Cotton swabs may contain certain fatty acids that can inhibit bacterial growth (Burns). Calcium alginate swabs can circumvent this problem, but this is not necessary, since inhibition is probably clinically insignificant. The lid margins are then wiped with a moistened applicator, and this also is streaked on the plate (Plate 45, Fig. 2). Both eyes should be cultured even though only one eye shows inflammation. In this way, bacteriologic findings can be compared between the normal and the diseased eye, since some pathogens may be present normally without producing disease, and so-called nonpathogens can cause disease. In normal eyes, the following bacteria are found in approximately these frequencies (Locatcher-Khorazo and Shegal)*:

Staphylococcus epidermidis	75–90%
Diphtheroids (eg, *Corynebacterium xerosis*)	20–33%
Staphylococcus aureus	20–25%
Alpha-hemolytic *Streptococcus*	2–6%
Haemophilus (children under 3)	3%
Pneumococcus	1–3%
Gram-negative rods	1%
Pseudomonas	0–5%

We prefer to use a method of streaking originally described by Dr. Phillips Thygeson of the Proctor Foundation (Plate 45, Figs. 3, 4).

As previously mentioned, eye cultures should be inoculated directly onto media rather than placed in a carrier because eye samples are small and often contain fastidious organisms. In a patient with unilateral conjunctivitis, the lacrimal system may be at fault. Anaerobic organisms may be the cause of the inflammation in cases of canaliculitis (actinomyces and others) and occasionally in dacryocystitis. In these cases, thioglycollate broth can be used conveniently, although it is not ideal for general anaerobes except actinomyces.

Suspected anaerobic specimens should be inoculated below the pink (aerobic) zone of the broth. If the pink zone is large, the broth can be boiled for a few minutes to expel oxygen. However, a much better broth for isolating general anaerobes is *chopped meat glucose* broth,

---

Note that bacterial populations may vary from region to region, and the above is meant as a guide.

which is more nutritional and maintains a reduced state longer than does thioglycollate. If the patient has been on antibiotics just immediately before being seen, a tube of enriched broth should also be inoculated routinely, since the broth in this case may show growth when solid medium may not.

Obtaining Lacrimal Canaliculus Specimen

This technique is particularly important when one is considering the diagnosis of canaliculitis. The conjunctiva is anesthetized, and a support such as an applicator or lid plate is put behind the canaliculus. Pressure is then applied anteriorly to express a specimen (Plate 45, Fig. 5). If large concretions or diverticuli are encountered, the canaliculus may have to be split. Once obtained, the concretions are crushed, saline is added, and smears are prepared. The smears are fixed in methanol and stained with gram and Giemsa stains. Specimens should be cultured in *anaerobic,* fungal, and aerobic media.

Obtaining Lacrimal Sac Specimens

It is important to express material from the lacrimal sac in the proper fashion. Secretions from the sac can be obtained by firm pressure over the sac fundus with an applicator stick while observing the lacrimal punctum, which has first been everted and cleansed (Plate 46, Fig. 1). In this way, even a scanty secretion will not be missed if it should roll into the fornix. It should be stressed that in suspected bacterial or fungal corneal ulcers, examination of the lacrimal sac contents must not be overlooked. Specimens should be smeared on slides for gram and Giemsa stains and cultured in aerobic, fungal, and anaerobic media.

CORNEAL ULCER WORK-UP

Laboratory investigation is imperative in the management of a bacterial or fungal corneal ulcer. This should be done for all corneal ulcers suspected of being bacterial or fungal before antibacterial or antifungal therapy is started. Once antibiotic therapy has been started, the yield from a microbiologic work-up is decreased markedly even though the infection may be ongoing. Once the necessary microbiologic work-up is done, a reasonable plan of antibiotic therapy can be initiated. The antibiotic regimen is modified, if necessary, after the exact organism has been identified and sensitivities determined. Bacteriologic or fungal cultures and smears are significant only when the result of the smear or culture is positive. If negative, this result alone does not absolutely rule out bacterial or fungal infection. In fact, a corneal biopsy may be needed to diagnose a fungal corneal ulcer when repeated cultures have been negative (Plate 46, Fig. 2). Cultures are, generally, the more sensitive means of establishing a diagnosis as compared to smears, although both should be done in the primary work-up.

The smear often gives prompt information which may be helpful in deciding on immediate therapy. The more common organisms responsible for corneal ulcers are as follows:

A. Bacterial
   1. *Staphylococcus*
   2. *Pseudomonas*
   3. *Streptococcus pneumoniae (pneumococcus)*
   4. *Moraxella*
   5. *Neisseria gonorrhoeae*
   6. *Streptococcus pyogenes*
   7. *Klebsiella pneumoniae*
   8. *Escherichia coli*
   9. *Proteus mirabilis*
   10. *Haemophilus influenzae* (less common)
   11. *Serratia marcescens* (less common)
   12. *Mycobacterium* spp (less common)

B. Fungal
   1. *Candida*
   2. *Aspergillus*
   3. *Fusarium* (especially *F. solani*)
   4. *Cephalosporium*
   5. *Penicillium*

We prefer to use the following material and techniques in a work-up for any corneal ulcer which is suspected of being bacterial or fungal. The conjunctiva and lid margins of the involved eye and the normal eye are cultured as above on blood agar, using the streaking technique recommended. Chocolate agar is also used routinely. (Plate 46, Fig. 3). Sabouraud's dextrose agar is used if a fungus is suspected, allowing suppression of bacterial growth because of hyperosmolality and poor nutrition for bacterial growth. No saprophytic inhibitor, such as cyclohexamide, should be present in the medium, since so-called nonpathogenic fungi often cause eye infections. It should be noted that fungi will grow on blood agar plates at room temperature if Sabouraud's agar is not available.

A sterile, dry, cotton-tipped applicator is then touched to the central area of the ulcer mainly to remove any superficial debris and exudate prior to scraping. This material is then streaked on the same blood agar plate that was used for the non-specific conjunctival cultures, using multiple C streaks. Following this, topical anesthetic is instilled. We prefer proparacaine to other topical anesthetics because it probably has the least bacteriostatic effect in this class of drugs. We wait for approximately five minutes after topical instillation of the anesthetic to minimize anesthetic presence. The ulcer is then scraped multiple times with our modification of the Kimura spatula at both the leading edge and the central deeper area (Plate 46, Fig. 4). The Kimura spatula is ideal for conjunctival scrapings, but not for corneal ulcers. The spatula is modified by us by tapering it to a more narrow tip and roughening the platinum surface and edge with a fine carborundum hone stone. The narrowed spatula is more useful for all size ulcer craters and is able to debride and hold corneal specimens much better than is the standard Kimura spatula (Plate 46, Fig. 5). We prefer to inoculate the microbiologic media before preparation of slides, since we feel that cultures are more specific and usually give a higher yield of positive results than does the gram stain when the patient has not previously been on antibiotics. *Multiple* scrapings are done, and the material obtained is *multiple C-streaked* directly onto the solid media. When streaked in this manner, any growth on a C streak is specific, while growth off a C streak is interpreted as probably contamination (Plate 47, Fig. 1).

Appropriate broths, including chopped meat glucose broth and Brewer's medium for anaerobes, are also inoculated directly. We then rescrape, using material to make at least two slides—one for the gram stain which is most important when a bacterial or yeast agent is suspected, and the other for a Giemsa stain to help rule out a fungal ulcer. Fungi will often stain with the gram stain, but the Giemsa stain will show the hyphate crosswalls better. Using specially prepared slides, a modified methenamine-silver stain as described by Forster may be more ideal for fungal stains (see section on stains). Also, wet preparations may demonstrate spore arrangement, helping to differentiate the fungus. The specimen is placed on a slide without distribution, potassium hydroxide is added, and the slide is flamed lightly to dissolve debris. If enough material is available, we routinely inoculate additional slides. These slides can be used for repeat gram stains, for Giemsa stains, for acid-fast stains, or for fungal stains. All slides are placed immediately in methyl alcohol for five minutes to allow fixation without loss of cellular structure before either gram or Giemsa staining. It is important to smear these slides firmly and evenly and to keep the smear as thin as possible.

Results from the cultures of the lids and conjunctiva and cultures of the dry swab that was used to clear the debris and exudate from the

Table 1.
MATERIALS REQUIRED FOR WORK-UP
OF A CORNEAL ULCER

1. Slit lamp or operating microscope
2. Anesthetic (proparacaine HCI, 0.5 percent is suggested, since it is less bacteriostatic than others)
3. Sterile cotton-tipped applicators—or calcium alginate swabs (Calgiswab, Colab Laboratories)
4. Kimura spatula (Storz E1091—modify the spatula as described in text). Before use, spatula is sterilized by flaming and, of course, cooled
5. Microbiologic media
   For bacterial ulcers: blood agar (two plates, one for lids and conjunctiva and one for ulcer itself), chocolate agar, brain-heart infusion broth (or other enriched broth as high-yield culture medium), and chopped meat glucose broth (helpful particularly for general anaerobes). For fungal ulcers: add Sabouraud's dextrose agar plate (without cyclohexamide, an inhibitor of saprophytic fungi)
6. Clean glass slides, coverslip for KOH mount; gelatin slide for GMS stain.
7. Methyl alcohol fixative—fix slides immediately after smearing
8. Stains
   A. Gram—for bacteria; sometimes useful for hyphae and yeast forms which stain gram-positive
   B. Giemsa—mainly for hyphae and yeast forms; better than gram stain for hyphae (Note that Giemsa stain may be useful for fungi but its main value is for cytology and inclusion bodies.)
   C. Acid-fast—*Mycobacterium and some Actinomyces*
   D. KOH wet preparation—hyphal fragments may be appreciated better after debris is digested by KOH
   E. Modified methenamine–silver stain–good for fungus smears as modified by Forster (see section on stains)

Table 2.
GRAM'S DIFFERENTIAL STAIN FOR BACTERIA

1. Fix the slide in methanol for five minutes or by gently flaming
2. Flood the slide with crystal violet. Rinse with water
3. Flood the slide with iodine.
4. Tilting the slide, allow the ethyl alcohol-acetone decolorizing solution to run over the slide until the purple color ceases to be washed off
5. Counterstain by flooding the slide with safranin. Rinse with water and gently blot dry

Each solution may be left on for a longer period of time (30 seconds) if you wish to preserve the slide (for teaching purposes, and so on). For routine clinical use, however, 1 to 3 seconds is sufficient time for the cells to become properly stained

ulcer are nonspecific. They may be helpful, however, in management decisions when the direct corneal cultures and slides are negative. By far the most important and most specific part of the ulcer work-up is the multiple C streaks made with the modified Kimura spatula. The required materials in a corneal ulcer work-up are summarized in Table 1, and gram stain procedure in Table 2. Our work-up sequence is schematically illustrated in Plate 47, Fig. 2. A good review by Jones of management of bacterial corneal ulcers has been published and should be reviewed.

ENDOPHTHALMITIS WORK-UP

In any case of suspected endophthalmitis, a microbiologic work-up is imperative. We routinely culture conjunctiva and lid margins of both eyes, as outlined above, on blood agar and Sabouraud's media. If there is any stitch abscess or infiltrate, this should also be cultured. This material should go onto both solid medium and into enriched broth.

In a case of suspected endophthalmitis, it is necessary to tap the anterior chamber to obtain aqueous samples (Allansmith et al). We do this after topical anesthesia. Some patients may require subconjunctival xylocaine near the area of the paracentesis. We feel that unless the wound is already gaping and can be conveniently entered, the paracentesis should be made through the corneal limbus inferotemporally. Fixation should be made at the site of entrance and not at 180 degrees from the entrance site, thereby producing less deformity of the globe. A rotary motion may be helpful in introducing the needle more easily. An assistant should aspirate while the surgeon controls fixation of the globe and the needle. A tuberculin syringe with a 27-gauge disposable needle is best, and 0.1 ml can usually be obtained. We prefer to already have 0.4 ml of enriched broth in the syringe before we enter the anterior chamber. This way we have a total of at least 0.5 ml of material which, after mixing in the syringe, is handled in the following manner:

One drop each is placed on a blood agar plate, a chocolate agar plate, and a Sabouraud's plate, one drop each is placed on four slides, and the remaining amount is injected into enriched broth and chopped meat glucose broth for general anaerobic culture. After immediately fixing all slides for five minutes in methyl alcohol, two slides are used for gram and Giemsa stains. Extra slides are stained as needed. The material on the solid media is streaked out.

Vitreous aspiration should be reserved for those cases with

definite vitreous involvement, penetrating trauma with introduction of material into the vitreous, and endogenous endophthalmitis. A vitreous tap may be positive when an anterior tap is negative (Forster, 1974). A vitreous tap should probably be done in the operating room if possible, whereas we have usually done anterior chamber taps in the minor surgery room. The technique we prefer for doing a vitreous tap is through a separate, small, 2 mm sclerotomy incision 4 mm posterior to the limbus through pars plana after a peritomy inferotemporally. The scleral incision is made to the deep scleral fibers without penetrating the latter. An 18- or 20-gauge disposable needle on a tuberculin syringe is usually adequate to obtain 0.4 to 0.5 ml of liquid vitreous. The material is handled in the same manner as the material in the anterior chamber tap.

In a case of suspected endophthalmitis, one should not start antibiotic therapy (even topical antibiotic therapy) until the appropriate microbiologic work-up is started. The feeling is almost universal that anterior chamber taps should be routine in cases of suspected endophthalmitis. However, not all authorities are in agreement with whether or not vitreous taps should also be done. We feel that they are indicated if, on immediate evaluation, the anterior chamber tap slide stains are negative microbiologically. If the slide stains show organisms (and the patient has not been on antibiotic therapy recently), the cultures will usually be positive. We do not routinely do a vitreous tap on a patient with a positive anterior chamber smear.

SMEARS AND SCRAPINGS OF THE CONJUNCTIVA

Slides may be prepared by swabbing exudate present in the conjunctival cul-de-sac or on the lid margin with a cotton-tipped applicator and spreading it on a clean glass slide. However, in most cases of bacterial conjunctivitis, recognizable organisms may not be seen in a smear of exudate, whereas a conjunctival scraping may more readily demonstrate them. The material is usually stained by Gram's method and observed under the microscope. When one suspects a neisserial infection in a purulent conjunctivitis, it is even more important to do a scraping of the infected conjunctival epithelium for early diagnosis. As the organisms are intracellular parasites, the intraepithelial gonococcus may be found before the smear exudate is positive. The material from the scraping should be spread in a thin layer on a clean glass slide and stained with gram stain. The gram stain is useless for giving any reliable information regarding cytologic response.

Scrapings of the conjunctiva should be taken from the site of maximum infection. Scraping is most valuable in the active phase of disease. If the upper tarsal conjunctiva is involved in the disease process, this is the ideal site from which to obtain conjunctival scrapings. The conjunctiva is first generally anesthetized with a topical anesthetic. After eversion of the upper tarsus, the tarsus is again anesthetized. The tarsal conjunctiva should then be lightly scraped with an unmodified platinum spatula which has been flamed and cooled (Kimura spatula, Storz E1091). This is an excellent spatula for conjunctival scrapings, cools quickly, and will last for decades. Material obtained by conjunctival scrapings using Bard-Parker or Beaver blades is usually unsatisfactory. The scraping is done mainly to remove surface cells and epithelium and should be away from the lid margin, which may normally contain keratinized cells. During the scraping sweep, the conjunctiva should be mildly blanched by the spatula (Plate 47, Fig. 3).

A scraping containing an excessive amount of blood is usually unsatisfactory and should be repeated. Such a scraping may harvest peripheral blood elements that may be misleading. Material should be visualized at the tip of the spatula and spread firmly and evenly in a thin layer on a clean glass slide (Plate 47, Fig.4). Slides prepared for gram staining should be fixed in methyl alcohol before staining or lightly flamed. Slides prepared for Giemsa staining must be immediately placed in methyl alcohol to prevent any drying effect and to preserve cytologic features (Plate 47, Fig. 5). Slides for Giemsa staining should not be flamed, since cytologic features will be altered. Slides prepared for Papanicolau staining (which may be useful in certain epithelial tumors or when searching for intranuclear inclusion bodies) should be immediately placed in an alcohol-ether solution to minimize drying and preserve cytologic features.

PARINAUD'S OCULOGLANDULAR SYNDROME WORK-UP

Parinaud's oculoglandular syndrome is now defined as a conjunctivitis with a variety of causative agents. Clinically the conjunctivitis is usually unilateral, with granulomatous nodules or vegetations (with or without ulceration and/or follicles) and regional lymphadenopathy. The causes of the syndrome may be bacterial, fungal, chlamydial, or other nonspecific agents (see Table 3). Details of the work-up can be found elsewhere (Hyndiuk and Chin). However, a practical guide to the work-up is given in Table 4.

Table 3.
CAUSES OF PARINAUD'S
OCULOGLANDULAR SYNDROME

USUALLY

1. Cat-scratch disease
2. Tularemia
3. Sporotrichosis

OCCASIONALLY

4. Tuberculosis
5. Syphilis
6. Coccidioidomycosis

RARELY

7. Chancroid
8. *Pasteurella multocida*
9. *Yersinia pseudotuberculosis*
10. Glanders
11. Listerellosis
12. Lymphogranuloma venereum
13. Actinomycosis
14. Blastomycosis
15. Infectious Mononucleosis

Table 4.
PRACTICAL APPROACH TO LABORATORY DIAGNOSIS
IN PARINAUD'S OCULOGLANDULAR SYNDROME

IMMEDIATE CONSIDERATION IN DIAGNOSIS

1. Culture: blood agar, broth (thioglycollate, brain-heart), Sabouraud's
2. Scrapings: gram, Giemsa, and acid fast stains
3. Serum sample (acute) for tularemia, syphilis, coccidioidomycosis (if skin test is positive), infectious mononucleosis
4. Skin tests
5. Medical consultation if indicated

LATER CONSIDERATIONS IF WARRANTED

1. CBC (cat-scratch disease, infectious mononucleosis)
2. Serum (convalescent) for tularemia, syphilis, coccidioidomycosis, infectious mononucleosis
3. Chest x-ray, (tuberculosis, coccidioidomycosis, blastomycosis, sarcoid, and glanders)
4. Biopsy
   a. Culture
   b. Histopathology
   c. Animal inoculation

OCULAR CYTOLOGY

The techniques for obtaining conjunctival scrapings have already been reviewed above. As a general rule, corneal scrapings are not valuable for cytology, except when the cornea is involved by a tumor, or in an occasional case of epithelial herpetic keratitis due to multiplying virus, when the diagnosis is clinically in doubt. A corneal scraping of active epithelial herpetic keratitis often demonstrates giant cells with the Giemsa stain. However this is usually a clinical diagnosis. In material stained by the Giemsa technique, it is rare to see intranuclear inclusions in herpes patients. These can be demonstrated better using a Papanicolau stain with an acid fixative. Remember that the tissue obtained from the scraping should be broken up into as thin a smear as possible for maximum visibility of individual cells. One should smear the slide firmly and evenly, thereby providing a thin smear.

STAINS IN OCULAR CYTOLOGY

Giemsa Stain.   Giemsa stain involves the 5-minute immediate fixation of the specimen in methyl alcohol, 60-minute incubation in fresh stain mixture at 37 C, and quick decolorization in ethyl alcohol.

1. Immediately fix the slide in methyl alcohol for at least 5 minutes. Do not air dry or flame.
2. Prepare a fresh stain solution for each batch of slides: mix stock Giemsa stain with a neutral buffer in a ratio of 1:20. Place the slide in the container (a coplin stain jar is recommended, since it can accommodate several slides and requires only 30 ml of diluted stain solution) and incubate at 37 C for 40 to 60 minutes
3. Rinse the slide quickly in ethyl alcohol. Air dry

To reiterate several important points:

1. The material should be spread firmly and evenly to provide a thin smear
2. Fixation should be in absolute methanol for at least 5 minutes
3. Fixation should be started immediately after smearing in order to prevent drying artifacts

Wright Stain.   Wright stain is done by air drying a thin smear, flooding the slide with the stain solution for 1 minute, adding distilled water so that the stain is diluted about one-half, and allowing it to react for 7 to 10 minutes. The slide is then rinsed with tap water. Note that the Wright stain is not satisfactory for ocular cytology. It may be the only one that certain hospitals are familiar with, but it is satisfactory only for demonstration of inflammatory cells.

A Rapid cytology stain (15 seconds) is also available. Solutions for the rapid stain are made by Harleco and available through Scientific Products Catalog (Harleco Diff-Quik Kit 64851).

Papanicolau Stain. A PAP stain is a complex staining procedure, involving incubation in several concentrations of various stains, xylene, and alcohols (see section on stains).

Hansel Stain. This is better than Giemsa or Wright stain for eosinophiles (see section on stains).

MISCELLANEOUS STAINS IN MICROBIOLOGY (LENNETTE ET AL)

Methylene Blue Stain

1. Fix the slide by passing it through the flame three or four times
2. Stain with methylene blue for five minutes
3. Wash with water
4. Dry, and examine under oil

The stain is especially suitable for *Pityrosporum ovale* in seborrheic blepharitis.

Acid-fast Stain (Ziehl-Neelsen)

1. Fix the slide by passing it through the flame three or four times
2. Apply Ziehl's carbolfuchsin solution
3. Gently steam the slide by careful heating for 3 to 5 minutes with intermittent replacement of the evaporating carbofuchsin solution
4. Wash with water
5. Decolorize with acid alcohol until only a slight suggestion of pink remains
6. Wash with water
7. Counterstain with Löffler's methylene blue for 30 seconds
8. Wash with water
9. Dry, and examine under oil

Capsule Stain (Hiss Method). The best source of material for the demonstration of capsules by this method is infected exudate. If a stock culture is to be examined, the organisms should be emulsified in a drop of serum on the slide.

Materials:
Gentian violet or fuchsin solution
Saturated alcoholic solution of gentian violet or
    basic fuchsin   5 ml
Distilled water   95 ml
Copper sulfate
    Copper sulfate   20 ml
    Water   100 ml

Technic:
1. The film is dried but not fixed with heat
2. Flood the glass slide with gentian violet or fuchsin solution
3. Hold the preparation for a second over a free flame until it steams
4. Wash off the dye with the copper sulfate solution (Do not wash with water)
5. Blot

Neisser Stain. For staining Klebs-Loffler bacilli and C. xerosis to show metachromatic granules. Use a 24 hour culture on blood serum. Make films and stain with methylene blue for one-half minute. Wash in tap water and treat with Bismarck brown for one-half minute. Wash, dry, and mount. The metachromatic granules stain very dark; the bodies light yellow.

1. Methylene blue (Neisser s)
    Methylene blue   1 g
    Alcohol, 96 percent   20 ml
    Glacial acetic acid   50 ml
    Water   950 ml
2. Bismarck brown
    Bismarck brown   1 g
    Water   100 ml

Papanicolaou Stain

Method:
1. Place specimen on a clean slide and immediately, without drying, fix in 95 percent ethanol
2. Remove slide from ethanol and place in parlodion for 1 minute
3. Transfer the slides without drying, from the parlodion,

to a slide carrier and sequentially to baths with 80 percent ethanol, another 80 percent alcohol and then to 50 percent ethanol, solutions, for 1 minute each; rinse with distilled water for 1 minute

4. Stain the slides in Mayer's Hematoxylin for 5 minutes, rinse in 3 successive baths of distilled water; the last bath also containing Lithium Carbonate (20 drops/900 ml), the slides should remain in the last bath for 2 minutes

5. Allow the slides to sit in a container with dripping water for 6 minutes and then drain

6. Run the slides up through 50 percent, 70 percent and 95 percent ethanol, leaving in each solution for approximately ½ minute each

7. Stain in Orange G-6 for 2 minutes

8. Rinse in two separate changes of 95 percent ethanol

9. Stain in EA-50 (Eosin) for 3 minutes

10. Rinse in 3 separate changes in 95 percent ethanol

11. Rinse successively in 100 percent ethanol, 100 percent ethanol, 100 percent ethanol/xylene, for 1 minute, 2 minutes and 2 minutes respectively

12. Rinse in 3 separate changes of xylene for 3 minutes each

13. Rinse in a final xylene solution for 10 minutes

14. Mount, without drying, using a coverslip

Epithelium cells appear as basophilic cells; the cytoplasm is semi-transparent and stains blue-green with the papanicolaou stain; the typical nucleus is dark blue, evenly distributed, with occasional small red, round prominent nucleoli.

Modified Grocott's Methenamine-Silver Nitrate Stain. This stain is used routinely for fungi in histopathologic sections. This procedure has been modified to reduce the two hour standard method to one hour for corneal scrapings for fungal identification (Forster, 1976).

Method:
1. Use slides that are coated with a film of gelatin to fix the specimens to the slide during staining procedure; this is done by placing a drop of warm gelatin (1 percent) and spreading it out to form a thin preparation; these may be stored in the freezer and used as needed

2. Spread the corneal scrapings on the gelatin slide very thinly

3. Fix the slide in methanol for 5 minutes

4. Oxidize the slide in 5 percent Chromic Acid for 30 minutes; prepare the working solution of Methenamine-Silver Nitrate
5. Pre-heat the working solution, in a water bath or an oven, to 58-60 c
6. Place the slide in the heated Methenamine-Silver Nitrate solution for 20 minutes, the smear will assume an amber color
7. When the amber color change has occurred, promptly discard the methanamine silver and wash the slide with six changes of distilled water by filling and emptying the staining jar with the distilled water
8. Tone for 2-4 minutes in 0.1 percent gold chloride; after use the gold chloride can be poured back into the stock jar
9. Rinse the slide with two changes of distilled water
10. Place slides in 2 percent thiosulfate for two minutes to remove reduced silver
11. Wash with tap water
12. Counter stain briefly with working light green solution (about 40 seconds)
13. Air dry and mount

Results: Stains fungus cell walls and septa black; the background is transparent green. For fungus the stain is more reliable than the KOH, Gram or Giemsa stain.

Solutions:
1. Methenamine Silver Nitrate Solution
   Solution A
   Borax 5 percent   8.0 ml
   Distilled water   100.0 ml
   Solution B
   Silver Nitrate, 10 percent   7.0 ml
   Methenamine, 3 percent   100.0 ml

Add equal parts of Solution A and B to make the working solution of Methenamine Silver Nitrate Solution. These should be made fresh each time.

2. Stock Light Green Solution
   Light green S.F. (yellow)   0.2 gm
   Distilled Water   100.0 ml
   Glacial Acetic Acid   0.2 ml

Hansel Stain (Excellent for eosinophiles)

1. Spread scrapings thinly on slide
2. Fix slide in methanol for 5 minutes
3. Cover slide completely with Hansel's stain and allow to stand for 30 seconds
4. Add distilled water and allow to stand for 30 seconds, pour off stain and flood slide with distilled water to remove excess stain
5. Flood slide with 95 percent ethyl or methyl alcohol, drain and dry in air

Eosinophiles with their red-staining granules stand out sharply with the contrasting blue color of the neutrophiles. Basophiles show both colors. Bacteria stain blue.
(Hansel stain: Lide Laboratories, Inc., 515 Timberwyck, St. Louis, Mo. 63131)

Lactophenol Cotton Blue Mounting Medium. This stain is used (in moist preparation) for fungi. It can be purchased ready-made.

1. Put a drop of this medium on the slide
2. Add specimen of fungus. Tease fungus with dissecting needle
3. Examine under a coverslip

It is hoped that the preceding outline will be of some direct practical value in helping the clinician arrive at a correct diagnosis via a current rational and systematic approach to office techniques. When applied properly, the laboratory methods can be a boon to both the patient and the physician in providing a better understanding and more rapid resolution of serious infections involving the eye.

ACKNOWLEDGMENTS

We thank Ms. Helane Neufeld and Ms. Barbara Morley, Milwaukee County Medical Complex, and Mas Okumoto, the Proctor Foundation, for their advice, Ms. Marianne Scannell for help in preparation of the manuscript, and Dr. R. Charlin and Mrs. Sue Sabin for help in preparing the illustrations. Many of the thoughts in this chapter were seeded or nurtured through associations with Drs. Herbert Kaufman, A.E. Braley, Phillips Thygeson, and Mas Okumoto.

REFERENCES

Allansmith MR, Skaggs C, Kimura SJ: Anterior chamber paracentesis. Arch Ophthalmol 84:745, 1970

Burns RP: Laboratory methods in diagnosis of eye infections. New Orleans Academy of Ophthalmology: Infectious Diseases of Conjunctiva and Cornea: Symposium. St. Louis, Mosby, 1963, pp 13–25

Forster RK: Endophthalmitis. Arch Ophthalmol 92:387, 1974

Forster RK: Methenamine-silver nitrate stained corneal scrapings in keratomycosis. Am J Ophthalmol 82:261–65, 1976

Hyndiuk RA, Chin GN: Parinaud's oculoglandular syndrome. In Duane T (ed): Clinical Ophthalmology. Hagerstown, Md, Harper and Row, in press

Jones DB: Early diagnosis and therapy of bacterial corneal ulcers. Int Ophthalmol Clin 13:1, 1973

Lennette EH, Spaulding EH, Truant JP: Manual of Clinical Microbiology, 2nd ed. Washington, DC, American Society for Microbiology, 1974

Locatcher-Khorazo D, Shegal BC: Microbiology of the Eye. St. Louis, Mosby, 1972

Index